Health care poli
the implicatio

Health care policies and Europe:

the implications for practice

Carole Ludvigsen, MA European Studies, BEd(Hons),
Cert Ed, SRN, RMN,
*Formerly Project Manager, European Opportunities Initiative at Hull
and Holderness Community Health NHS Trust; European Officer,
Northern and Yorkshire Regional Health Authority*

Kathleen Roberts, BA(Hons), PGCE
*Consultant and Freelance writer; formerly European Officer, North
Yorkshire Local Education Authority and Leeds City Council*

Foreword by:
The Right Honourable Sir Leon Brittan QC
Vice-President of The European Commission

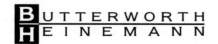

BUTTERWORTH
HEINEMANN

Butterworth-Heinemann
Linacre House, Jordan Hill, Oxford OX2 8DP
A division of Reed Educational and Professional Publishing Ltd

Ǫ A member of the Reed Elsevier plc group

OXFORD   BOSTON   JOHANNESBURG
MELBOURNE   NEW DELHI   SINGAPORE

First published 1996

British Library Cataloguing in Publication Data
A catalogue record for this book is available from the British Lihrary.

Library of Congress Cataloguing in Publication Data
A catalogue record for this book is available from the Library of Congress.

ISBN 0 7506 2485 X

Photoset by Wilmaset Ltd, Birkenhead, Wirral
Printed and bound in Great Britain by Biddles Ltd,
Guildford and King's Lynn

Contents

Foreword

I am happy to be able to commend this book on Europe and health. The authors have seen the need for a wide variety of professionals to be aware of European activities and legislation and have responded to that need by producing a guide for the health sector.

Such initiatives are essential. European legislation today affects an enormous variety of areas of everyday life. As this book shows, the European Union may have a limited formal competence in public health matters, but health professionals are concerned not just with this, but with the operation of the internal market, with professional mobility and exchange programmes, with the challenges that we face at European level. Indeed it is only when one reads a text such as this that the extent of professional concerns emerge.

Perhaps most important of all is Chapter 9 'How to influence the European agenda'. The European institutions are in their nature very open – often far more open than the Civil Services of Member States. This is a recognition of the need for an input by each sector, and the added value which such inputs bring. I hope that those who read this book will be encouraged to put their point of view across, and to use their influence and authority to ensure that the activities in the health field are well designed and bring genuine added value to what can be achieved nationally.

The Right Honourable Sir Leon Brittan, QC,
Vice-President of the European Commission

Biographical details of authors

Carol Ludvigsen and Kathleen Roberts met on a visit to Brussels, when they were both working as European Officers, and have since collaborated on various European projects and initiatives.

Carol has considerable experience of working within the UK health service, as a nurse and nurse tutor, and as European Officer for the Northern and Yorkshire Regional Health Authority. More recently, she was Project Manager, European Opportunities Initiative, at Hull and Holderness Community Health NHS Trust. Carol moved to France in April 1996 and now lives in the Limousin.

Kathleen worked in the education service for several years, both as an FE lecturer and in educational administration, before becoming a European Officer, first at Leeds City Council and later with the North Yorkshire Local Education Authority. She is now a consultant and freelance writer, and divides her time between North Yorkshire and a home in Lower Normandy.

ACKNOWLEDGEMENTS

The authors wish to thank the following: all those who contributed their views and experiences and whose names appear in the text; those long-suffering friends and colleagues who read and commented upon early drafts, most notably May Burden, Jonathan Hauxwell, Ian Hirst, Peter Horton, Mary Ness and Eugene O'Callaghan; Michael Scannell of the Cabinet of Commissioner Padraig Flynn; and our editor, Susan Devlin.

1

Introduction – How to use this book effectively

About the book

This book sets out to achieve a number of broad objectives. It aims to **inform** health and social care professionals about the European Union and its health-related policies and activities, to **explain** some of its complexities, and to **provide resources** to point readers in the direction of finding out more for themselves. It aims to **stimulate** interest in Europe, past, present and future, and it also aims to **challenge** some of the attitudes and preconceptions readers may have developed about Europe and question how these have arisen.

The book has been written in response to a developing European health and social agenda. No longer can health and social care professionals think and operate within a purely national consciousness: they, and the citizens they serve, are part of a European Union which numbers fifteen Member States and will grow yet larger and more culturally diverse. To retain our insularity within this setting is to risk isolation, both personally and professionally.

You may have bought this book because it is required reading for a course of education or training which has a newly-introduced European dimension. We are conscious that most health and social care professionals have to read enough dry and dusty textbooks during training, and we feel that this should be a pleasant read. No-one could turn a book on the subject of the European Union into a frivolous pot-boiler, but if Europe itself is an interesting place, why should a book about it be boring? (Though we defy anyone to produce fascinating descriptions of the workings of the European institutions.) Alternatively, you may have bought the book because you are considering working in another European country or, as an employer, recruiting practitioners trained in another Member State. You may be a tutor in further or higher education in need of accessible material and resources for one of your courses. Or perhaps you are simply interested in finding out about professional practice in other parts of the EU or exchanging ideas with European colleagues. These are all concerns which have been raised with us over the last year and which provided the original impetus for the writing of *Health Care Policies and Europe*. We believe that the timing of this book is crucial in enabling present and future practitioners to maximize the opportunities presented through membership of the Union.

The book's title reflects the fact that the health of the Union is a matter for concern for each of us, as individuals, as practitioners, as employees or employers. Awareness of *current* issues, trends and policies Europe-wide is essential if we are to be able to meet the challenge of *future* demands and opportunities. Issues such as the ageing population, social exclusion, the effects of long-term unemployment, environmental problems, the speed and diversity of technological advances, rising expectations and costs are pan-European concerns and we may hope for European solutions to some of them. We should also remember that we have an important and active part to play in creating and shaping the European Union of the future, and cannot afford to lack essential knowledge or adopt a passive stance.

The book is also written from a consciously pro-European stance: our views have been formed by several years of working within a European context and we want to be open about them – even if our readers don't agree with us. However, this is not a piece of propaganda, and we don't expect readers to undergo lightning conversions to our way of thinking. We just want them to think for themselves, and draw their own conclusions based on a knowledge of the subject and familiarity with the issues involved.

Because we think that Europe is a union of people, not just Member States, we have emphasized the personal as opposed to the institutional wherever possible. In certain chapters, we have focused on individual politicians, civil servants, practitioners and citizens and tried to express their views accurately and fairly. It is worth remembering, however, that they are often speaking for themselves and that their views should not be taken as representative of their countries or professions.

Using the book

Although the book is intended to be read as a whole, each chapter can be read as a self-contained unit if necessary. Chapters 2 and 3 summarize the history and evolution of the European Union and describe its institutions and the way they work. Many practitioners will find that the material here is not of direct relevance to their work, and may be tempted to skip them, and head straight for Chapter 4. If you do this, we recommend that you try to read the initial chapters at some stage because if you omit them completely you will lack fundamental knowledge about how the EU works and how it originated.

To help you to get the most out of the book and to home in on the issues and topics that interest you most, we have set out the aims of each chapter clearly at the start and provided 'Summary Points' for them which sum up the essential facts. Some recommendations may also be made on further reading. The final section of the book is a resource section, which contains information on the European Commission and Parliament, on useful contacts and sources of information, including publications, and there is also a short glossary of terms and 'Eurojargon'.

2

The evolution of the European Union

Aims of this Chapter

In this chapter, we aim to:
- explain the origins of the European Union;
- provide factual information about membership;
- introduce some technical terms and concepts which will be used subsequently throughout the book.

The Evolution of the European Union

At the end of the Second World War, Europe was in chaos. Economies had been devastated or bled dry by years of warfare, and the beginning of the Cold War was a reminder that hostility between nations was possible even in the aftermath of a major conflict which had cost millions of lives.

Against this backdrop, two Frenchmen worked together on a proposal which, with hindsight, was revolutionary in its simplicity and vision. Robert Schuman, the French Foreign Minister, and Jean Monnet, a civil servant, proposed that Germany and France should put aside their traditional antagonism and work collaboratively. On 9 May 1950, with an uneasy peace threatening to give way to a third world war, Schuman read out a declaration which stated:

> World peace cannot be safeguarded without creative efforts equal to the dangers which exist to world peace. By the

pooling together of basic production processes and the setting up of a new High Authority whose decisions will link France, Germany and the other countries which will accede, this proposal will bring to pass the first concrete steps of a European federation which is indispensable to the preservation of peace.

Initially, the joint action would be limited to collaboration on the production of coal and steel, important industries to both nations. Control would be placed under neither government, but under a separate High Authority with the power to make and implement decisions which would be binding on both. Schuman and Monnet also foresaw that other states would perceive the benefit of joining this community, and Italy, Belgium, the Netherlands and Luxembourg immediately proved them right. Thus was the first of the European Communities born, the European Coal and Steel Community (ECSC), established in 1951.

In 1957, two more treaties were signed in Rome, establishing the European Atomic Energy Community (Euratom) and the European Economic Community (the EEC). (Thus the official title of the European Commission is 'The Commission of the European *Communities*', which refers to the fact that there are actually three.) In the latter treaty, the six nations agreed on a further stage of co-operation and partnership, in the form of a customs union. This committed them to an open market for goods produced throughout this economic area, with producers and manufacturers being free to trade without fear of protectionism from individual governments. This was the basis of the 'four freedoms': freedom of movement of goods, capital, services and people.

This was the state of affairs when the UK applied to join in 1961, along with Ireland and Denmark. The following year, Norway applied for membership. However, negotiations with all the applicants came to an abrupt halt in 1963 when President de Gaulle of France vetoed the UK application. Apparently, he feared that the UK would challenge the centre-stage role of France and the Franco-German alliance at the heart of the new Communities, and was also suspicious of Britain's close ties with the United States and its influence.

A further application in 1967 was again blocked by the French, and it was not until 1973 that the UK finally became a member of the European Community, in company with Ireland and Denmark. Norway held a referendum which resulted in a majority opposing membership. In 1981, Greece became a member, followed by Spain and Portugal in 1986. The Member States now numbered twelve, and the emblem of the EC became a circle of twelve stars (which it will remain despite the subsequent and future enlargement of the Union).

However, the free trade area envisaged when the EEC came into being was not established, and in practice, governments continued to keep barriers in place in order to protect their own industries. The 'Common Market' originally envisaged had simply failed to materialize due to lack of genuine commitment from all Member States. By the 1980s, it was recognized that the EEC had lost its momentum and that a new initiative was needed to redefine the European Community and to give it fresh impetus.

The lack of enthusiasm exhibited by Member State governments forced the European Commission's role onto centre-stage. In 1985, Jacques Delors, as president of the European Commission, presented a programme of measures intended to achieve an internal market for the European Community. Later that same year, the European Commission published a White Paper drawn up under the supervision of the British Commissioner Lord Cockfield, and entitled *Completing the Internal Market*. The White Paper set out 300 proposals (eventually reduced to 279) aimed at removing barriers to free movement of goods, services, people and capital – the so-called 'four freedoms'. The proposals formed the basis of the Single European Act of 1986, ratified by all 12 Member States and in force by 1 July 1987.

The deadline agreed for completion of the Single Market was 31 December 1992. For this reason, it was known as the '1992' programme, although the effective date was in fact 1 January 1993. By that date, 95 per cent of the relevant legislation had been passed, though obviously much of it was not in force at Member State level. The delays mainly centred on social legislation and the free movement of people, on which issues it had become apparent that there were major differences in interpretation. On the one hand, the European Commission and the Parliament shared the view that the ultimate goal should be a Europe without internal frontiers or customs checks, within which European citizens should be able to move freely. Social legislation was therefore seen to be essential to protect citizens and promote their well-being. Member State governments, on the other hand, were more cautious in their enthusiasm and the UK government, in particular, felt that European legislation should be limited to issues relating to economic concerns. Legal competence on issues relating to social rights for citizens should be left to national governments. This fundamental opposition came to a head with the adoption of a Charter on Fundamental Social Rights for Workers by 11 Member States in December 1989, the UK being the only State to opt out. The result was that when the Union treaty was drawn up, the UK refused to be a signatory because it objected to the inclusion of a Social Chapter. Consequently, the offending material was removed and formed the basis of a separate Social Protocol, which was agreed by the other 11 Member States, with the UK again abstaining from this. (In fact, the UK has subsequently implemented several of the proposals which arose from the Social Chapter, though it has also been instrumental in delaying or diluting the force of others.)

This latest European Treaty, the Treaty of European Union, was signed at Maastricht in February 1992, and is popularly known for this reason as 'The Maastricht Treaty'. It was necessary because the Community had developed to a degree where joint action was desirable in a range of areas where the EC had no legal competence. In addition, the democratic mechanisms and processes of the EC were felt to be weak. The Treaty therefore extended the scope and competence of previous legislation and began the process of laying a foundation for far-reaching social legislation at European level. It addressed what had been known as 'the democratic deficit' at European level by establishing a committee of democratically-elected regional representatives, the 'Committee of the Regions', and giving new powers to the European Parliament. The establishment of the Committee of the Regions was the cause of some controversy in the UK, with the Government initially appearing to take the view that members of the Committee could be nominees rather than elected representatives. The local authorities objected strongly to this, fearing that officials from regional offices of government departments or members of quangos would take up the UK seats. In the event, the membership was drawn from local and county council elected members.

This Committee now plays an important role in the EU legislative process, strengthening the democratic principle. It also provides a voice for Europe's regions and acknowledges their diversity. Most large European Member States, other than the UK, have some form of regional government, and the idea of a European institution based upon regional representation was not problematic for their national governments – indeed, it seemed a natural development at EU level which mirrored the national scene. In the UK, many local authorities feel they have found a more sympathetic ear at Brussels than at Westminster, and welcome opportunities for direct contact and influence. With so much power in Britain vested in central government, MPs and civil servants have no experience of real power-sharing and regard direct communication between Town Hall and Brussels as a bypassing of the Westminster power base, which many find threatening.

The Union Treaty emphasized the need for Member States to work collaboratively and to establish closer co-operation between governments in order to bring about improvements and raise standards across a range of policy areas. The Treaty also opened up new areas for EU activity including education, consumer protection and health. The Public Health Article of the Treaty is a recognition of the many common problems facing Member States and third countries (i.e., external to the EU), such as the fight against disease, the implications of an ageing population and the social impact of economic recession.

The concept of European citizenship was also given substance, with implementation focused on the need to create an awareness of European citizenship as an added dimension to an individual's national citizenship.

The Union Treaty contained a number of other fundamental changes, including those relating to closer economic and monetary union and foreign policy. These proved particularly controversial, and yet they were not intended to be goals in their own right but rather stages on a road that would ultimately lead even further (a uniform European foreign policy would inevitably make Europe an extremely powerful force on the world stage, but the implications, in terms of military co-operation, for example, are considerable.) However, they proved to be more like stumbling blocks than stepping stones and the economic recession affecting the EU exacerbated the problem. Member States meet again at an inter-governmental conference (IGC) in 1996 to take new decisions in light of the advances made in the period of 1993–96. This IGC has the potential to be an extremely significant event, with a high profile likely for social policy areas.

Despite the difficulties besetting the EU, Member States like France and Germany are committed to the 'ever-closer union' indicated in the Treaty and do not seem to fear a loss of sovereignty or erosion of their own national cultures. (In fact, the French in particular perceive the latter threat to emanate from the other side of the Atlantic, and worry about being swamped by American culture. Strangely, this is never mentioned in the UK, the European country where it is most evident.) The UK is not invariably the dissenting voice in Europe, but it seems to be the one country which lacks real commitment to maintaining the momentum of European Union, at least at the time of going to press.

Enlargement

Notwithstanding the difficulties being experienced by some governments in membership of the EU, other countries have been eager to join. In January 1995, Finland, Austria and Sweden became members, though Norway's membership was again blocked by the result of a referendum. Enlargement will continue, and the European Union of the future is likely to include a number of the countries of central and eastern Europe in due course. As the EU grows, it inevitably has the potential to be a more potent force on the world scene and a more powerful economic bloc, as well as an enormously

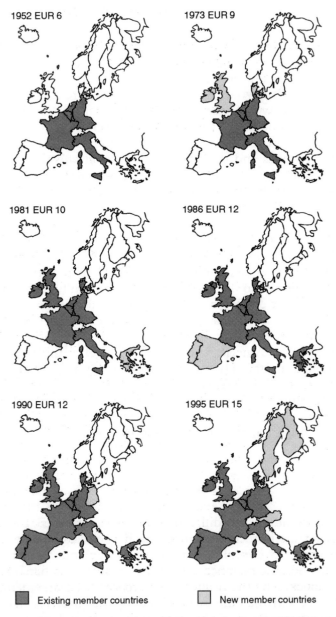

Figure 1 Maps of the European Union showing when countries joined. *Scource: The Institutions of the European Union.* (1995). *Europe on the Move* Series. Reproduced with kind permission of the Commission of the European Communities.

lucrative market. Those European countries outside it risk isolation and increasing economic vulnerability.

The status of the European Union and the principle of subsidiarity

As a body founded by international treaties, the European Union is a creation of law. It is also the source of a body of autonomous law that applies directly to the Member States and to individual citizens. However, laws are only made at European level when there is good reason, and where the European institutions have legal competence. This is the basis of the principle of subsidiarity: decisions should be taken as near to the citizen as possible. In other words, decisions will only be taken at EU level where this would be more effective than at Member State level alone.

Those who have been mystified by the heated arguments over sovereignty in the Westminster Parliament will wonder what all the fuss is about. Our politicians applied for membership of the 'Common Market', they were involved in the shaping of the European Union and they have been signatories to all the legislation which has created the current scenario. They were aware that power is a finite commodity; any government which invests another body or organization with powers which have previously been its own, inevitably diminishes its own authority. European law is directly binding on individuals living in the EU and takes precedence over national law. This does not necessarily mean a lessening of power for individual citizens, many of whom feel they have little or no influence on national policies anyway. But it does mean a reduction in the authority of politicians in national governments, for which surprisingly they seem to have been unprepared. As indicated earlier, governments in the UK (of whatever political hue) have not been accustomed to sharing power or to a model of partnership in government and administration. Over recent years, the British electorate has witnessed the reluctance of politicians at Westminster to relinquish any degree of their influence in the decision-making process. This has manifested itself both in the stance of

Ministers who have vetoed or diluted European legislation, and in the behaviour of back-benchers who would like to see the EU as nothing more than a free trade area.

European institutions are frequently said to have too much power. The UK tabloid press are not the only ones to make this allegation: British politicians can be heard on programmes such as Radio 4's respected *Today* talking about 'limiting the power of Brussels'. Many listeners may take these remarks at face value and infer that the European institutions do hold the balance of power, with Member State governments powerless to resist their headlong rush towards total economic and political union. In fact, the institution holding the real power in Europe is the Council of Ministers, which consists of ministers from the 15 Member States meeting in closed session. Until recently, documents such as minutes of meetings and other material have not been available to journalists or EU citizens, though this is likely to change in the future. The next chapter deals in more detail with the European institutions and should enable readers to draw some informed conclusions of their own.

European Union – something to celebrate?

The historic statement made by Robert Schuman on 9 May 1950 was remembered during the Milan Summit of 1985, when the European Heads of State and Government decided to commemorate that date as 'Europe Day'. According to the blurb provided by the Commission, it has been selected as 'the day to celebrate that the peoples of Europe co-operate in order to create peace and solve common problems'. Not surprisingly, most people are unaware of the designation.

Summary points

1 The European Community or Union is not a fixture (fixed entity). It has evolved gradually over a period of time from comparatively limited origins, in response to Western Europe's political, economic and social needs and aspira-

tions. Its further growth, shape and extent have still to be determined by the interaction of political will, public opinion and force of events. Its future is our future, and lies in our hands.

2 Evolution has meant a broadening of limits:
- From primary resources like, coal, steel and atomic energy to international trade.
- From trade and economic considerations to social aspects of European citizenship.
- From power vested in Councils of Ministers and Commissioners to more democratic representation and a voice for the people of Europe.
- From participation by Member State governments to access for their regions.
- From 6 members to 12 members to 15 members, with more to come.

3 There is a lot of myth and misconception surrounding the Union.

Further reading

Budd A. and Jones A. (1994). *The European Community: A Guide to the Maze*, 5th edn. Kogan Page.

Borchardt, Dr. K. D. (1995). *European Integration – the Origins and Growth of the European Union*. European Commission, Office for Official Publications of the European Communities.

3

The institutions of the European Union and how they work

Aims of this Chapter

In this chapter, we aim to:
- explain how the main European institutions work and interact;
- provide some personal insights into the institutions from people involved;
- explain the process of decision-making at EU level and how European legislation relates to national laws;
- briefly summarize the main points of the Maastricht Treaty;
- demystify some of the jargon and technicalities and debunk some of the myths which have grown up around the EU.

The European Union's institutions

The European Commission

The impression given by the British media is that the European Commission is a huge bureaucracy, staffed by faceless pen-pushing Eurocrats who wield mysterious and far-reaching powers, and seem to have it in for our best-loved British traditions. Hungry for even greater authority, they are building a vast power base in Brussels which will ultimately reduce the British government to a mere cipher, and the Palace of Westminster to a second-rate tourist attraction. The reality is rather more prosaic. The Commission is headed by the Commissioners themselves, who are proposed by their Member States and are usually senior politicians. Each is allocated a portfolio which is implemented by the Directorates General of the Commission (the 'DGs'). There are 24 DGs in total, and between them they are responsible for a diverse and heavy workload. The staffing establishment of the Commission is actually much smaller than that of many UK local authorities, though admittedly the ranks of Commission officials are also swelled by national government secondees. The officers working within the DGs, far from being faceless Eurocrats, are more easily accessible than civil servants of most national governments. (The authors have yet to meet a single Sir Humphrey amongst them.) Meetings with officials can be relatively easily arranged (always providing there is a genuine reason for them) and all dealings with the Commission are generally marked by a refreshing lack or formality and stuffiness.

The powers of the European Commission itself are limited, and are clearly defined by treaty. It can put forward new ideas for policy formation and implementation, but does not fix the overall future direction of policy. That is decided at the highest political level within the European Council (summit) of EU leaders and put into operation by the Council of Ministers, which is the most powerful of the EU institutions and the one which to date has been the least open.

The Commission's remit is threefold. In its **political** role, it makes policy proposals in line with agreed policy direction, and puts them to the Council of Ministers, where it will explain and defend them. This includes major initiatives such as reform of the Common Agricultural Policy, draft guidelines for negotiating with countries outside the EU, new research programmes for the Union, and detailed measures to create a single market for goods and services. It draws up a preliminary draft budget for the Union each year, which must go to the Council of Ministers and the European Parliament to be agreed. It also negotiates on behalf of the Union in international bodies like the GATT (General Agreement on Tariffs and Trade); and wherever the EU has economic relations with other countries, such as Japan, the United States, countries in the developing world and the states of Central and Eastern Europe. The Commission also has a **technical** role: it manages Union policies. For example, it administers the Union's funds for training, regional development and research, runs the common agricultural policy on a day-to-day basis and is responsible for carrying out assistance programmes for developing countries and states of Central and Eastern Europe. The Commission's **judicial** role is essential to the functioning of the Union; it must ensure that Member States implement EC laws once they have been agreed and see that they do not introduce measures which hamper the free movement of goods, services, capital and people between member countries.

The Commission must also ensure fair competition. It has to clamp down on unfair subsidies in one country which could undermine companies and jobs in other Member States and to ensure that firms are not 'carving up' the market through cartels or monopolies. This is a key role in the realization of the Single European Market.

The present Commission

The 20 members of the Commission are drawn from the 15 EU countries: the UK, France, Spain, Italy and Germany have two nominees each, the smaller nations one. Each Commissioner has been selected by his or her country but swears an oath of independence, ensuring that his or her allegiance is to the European Union as a whole, rather than one Member State.

The current President of the Commission is Jacques Santer, a former Prime Minister of Luxembourg and past Governor of both the International Monetary Fund and the European Bank for Reconstruction and Development. He succeeded Jacques Delors, frequently the butt of British tabloid rage and ridicule, but actually a very hard act to follow. Delors was not only a thoroughly committed European, but a very able and hard-working politician who was prepared to do battle for his beliefs – one of which was that the European Union must have a social dimension, in fairness to its citizens. Santer was originally perceived as a softer option than other pro-federalist candidates for the Presidency, but it remains to be seen whether this is a fair assessment of him.

The work of the Commission is divided into portfolios which are shared out between the Commissioners (jokingly referred to as 'Santer's little helpers' by one European journal). For example, Sir Leon Brittan shares the External Relations portfolio with his Spanish colleague Manuel Marin. The other UK Commissioner, Neil Kinnock, has responsibility for Transport issues.

(For more detail on the Commission, see the Factsheet on it in the Resource section at the end of the book.)

The Commission's year plan

Every year the Commission sets out its proposals for action in a year plan which is published, in line with its commitment to openness. The Commission (as well as the Parliament) also seeks advice from various Standing Committees which have been established for this purpose. (Health care personnel are elected to represent their country across a range of Committees representing all professional groups.) Additionally, each separate DG also announces its programme for the forthcoming year.

The Directorates General responsible for health issues

Currently there is no one single unit within the European Commission overseeing the totality of this work and different Directorates General are involved in different aspects of public health and health-related activities. The lead is generally taken by DGV (Public Health and Safety), but the others involved include DGs VIII (Development – which has a health and AIDS section), XI (Environment, Nuclear Safety and Civil Protection), XII (Science, Research and Development) and

XIII (Exploitation of Research and also telematics for health). DGV is split between Brussels and Luxembourg.

There may well be changes within the structure of the Commission in order to 'streamline' this area of activity and ensure more effective co-ordination and consultation. In 1994, a question was asked of the European Parliament about co-ordination of public health-related activity and the reply indicated an awareness on the part of the Commissioner concerned that changes might need to be made in order to respond adequately to the additional responsibility posed by Article 129 of the Union Treaty. This has been addressed largely by setting up internal networks between the DGs and strengthening the role of DGV's Directorate F, whose Public Health and Safety at Work portfolio includes implementation of the various disease-specific programmes, health promotion and disease surveillance, occupational health and hygiene and accidents and injuries at work. To facilitate and improve co-ordination of effort, an Interservice Group was set up by DGV to liaise with other Directorates General on health-related issues, and an assessment carried out by the relevant DGs. A report on the health protection requirements in Community policies was produced by the Commission (published as COM (95) 196 final) and presented to the appropriate European institutions. There has been some pressure from various groups for the appointment of a Commissioner for Health, but this does not seem likely in the foreseeable future.

The Commission has also demonstrated a willingness to co-operate with other groups which share its objectives, particularly on provision of information and consultation with the public. For example, it supported an initiative by the European Public Health Alliance (EPHA), a lobbying and umbrella group representing health care organizations and agencies, which set up a Health Hotline for four days during May 1995. EPHA was also assisted by the Euro Citizen Action Service. The Hotline provided an information service for enquirers all over Europe and also enabled people to raise issues and concerns on health-related matters. Hotline staff were apparently inundated by calls from all over the EU, even though the mass media had accorded little publicity to the initiative.

The Council of Ministers

The Council is the main legislative arm of the Union and has the last word on adopting EU law. As the European institutions now stand, it is the most powerful group in terms of decision-making. It brings together Ministers from each of the Member States for Council meetings, either in Brussels or Luxembourg. The Ministers who attend are those dealing with the subjects under discussion, so Fisheries Ministers would attend a Fisheries Council, Transport Ministers a Transport Council and so on.

In the light of the ongoing debate in the UK on the perceived powers of 'Brussels', it would appear that most citizens are unaware of the role of the Council of Ministers in the legislative process. The fact is that the ultimate decisions which bind Member States and create EU law are not made by the European Commission, nor yet by the Parliament. They are made by the representatives of Member State governments, trying to reach agreement with each other. Each state has a number of votes based on population (France, Germany and the UK have 10 each, the largest number). The total number of votes is 87 and a 'qualified majority' of 62 is needed for agreement (a 'blocking minority' of only 26 votes is needed to stop legislation). In practice, most important decisions are taken on the basis on unanimity.

Given this scenario, if a British government minister is unable to agree with his or her colleagues in the Council, it is not 'Brussels' he or she is holding out against, but the view of the other governments. Where 14 other States, representing a variety of shades of political opinion, have managed to find common ground with each other and the UK has disagreed and forced a rethink, this cannot, therefore, accurately be represented as a victory against the encroaching power of the European Commission.

Twice a year, the heads of state meet in a summit as the European Council.

Presidencies

The Council presidency rotates on a six-monthly basis between member countries. The Member State presiding will usually announce the priorities it has designated for its own presidency period and the objectives it seeks to achieve. The Presidencies are to run as follows:

1996 Italy and Ireland
1997 Netherlands and Luxembourg
1998 United Kingdom and Austria
1999 Germany and Finland
2000 Portugal and France
2001 Sweden and Belgium
2002 Spain and Denmark
2003 Greece

The Committee of Permanent Representatives (COREPER)

Each Member State has a permanent representative in Brussels, with an office staffed by diplomats who meet together in the Committee of Permanent Representatives. (The UK office is known as 'UK Rep'.) It prepares the way for ministerial meetings by resolving outstanding technical problems and identifies the political differences for Ministers to tackle. The negotiations usually focus on a proposal from the Commission, which can explain and defend its ideas during the proceedings and help to secure agreement around the table. If issues can be hammered out to the satisfaction of all those involved, discussions at the Council of Ministers are likely to go much more smoothly.

The European Parliament

The European Parliament does not have the same legislative role and functions as a national parliament, and its powers are considerably less. This gave rise to the concern that there was a 'democratic deficit' at European level, because the two institutions holding the most power – the Council of Ministers and the Commission – had not been democratically elected to this role by the citizens of Europe. (The Council is made up of Member State ministers who are usually, but not invariably, elected representatives, but inevitably operate from a national rather than pan-European stance.) The Union Treaty attempted to address this deficit, by giving more powers to the Parliament and also establishing a Committee of the Regions, comprising elected regional representatives.

The Parliament's powers are various and were extended under the Union Treaty. A new Commission is subject to a Parliamentary vote of approval before its Commissioners can take up office. When the current Commissioners were nominated in 1994, Parliament decided to give them a public grilling in order to ensure that they were fit for the job. They appeared before the main Parliamentary Committee relating to their portfolio, and all agreed to do this even though not obliged to do so by law. In fact, the Parliament could not actually reject any one Commissioner; it can only reject the whole Commission as a body (i.e. the college of Commissioners). It can sack the Commission by a two-thirds vote comprising an overall majority of its members, though it has never yet done so, and the circumstances which would justify such a move would be difficult to imagine. Relationships between the Parliament and the Commission tended to be stable throughout the last three Parliamentary terms, largely due to the respect accorded former Commission President Jacques Delors.

Another of Parliament's powers is to scrutinize Community legislation, using the committee system mentioned above. Each new proposal is forwarded to the Parliament, which designates one of its committees to work on it, examining the text, questioning the Commission and other interested parties, producing a report and usually proposing amendments. These amendments are then voted in plenary session. The Commission must decide whether to modify its own proposals in the light of the amendments which are passed. (See Figure 3 illustrating the decision-making process in the section on *How decisions are made*: it is not very straightforward, unfortunately, but neither is the process itself!)

The Parliament shares responsibility with the Council of

EUROPEAN PARLIAMENT: 626 members*

Parliament is presided over by a President assisted by 14 Vice-Presidents.

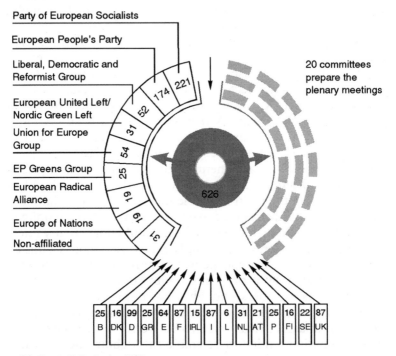

Party of European Socialists

European People's Party

Liberal, Democratic and
Reformist Group

European United Left/
Nordic Green Left

Union for Europe
Group

EP Greens Group

European Radical
Alliance

Europe of Nations

Non-affiliated

20 committees
prepare the
plenary meetings

221 174 52 31 54 25 19 19 31

626

25	16	99	25	64	87	15	87	6	31	21	25	16	22	87
B	DK	D	GR	E	F	IRL	I	L	NL	AT	P	FI	SE	UK

* Situation on 21 September 1995

Figure 2   The political breakdown of the European Parliament. *Source*:
Adapted from *The Institutions of the European Union.* (1995). *Europe on the
Move* Series. Reproduced with kind permission of the Commission of the
European Communities.

Ministers for the EU budget, with scope to amend and increase
spending plans within certain limits. Parliament can reject the
whole budget if agreement cannot be reached with the Council.
An overall majority of Parliament members must give its
approval to agreements with non-Union countries before they
can take effect. The Parliament also can formally question both
the Commission and the Council, with a question time at the
plenary sessions and a procedure for written questions.

The European Parliament guarantees participation of the people and exercises powers of democratic control. It conducts its work in the 11 official languages of the European Union, using simultaneous translation facilities. Debates are open to the public, and students in particular are encouraged to visit the Parliament buildings in both Brussels and Strasbourg and see MEPs in action.

The European Parliament is presently composed of 626 MEPs (Figure 2). In the Chamber, Members are not grouped in national delegations but according to the political group to which they belong. (These are inevitably rather broad alignments.)

The largest group is the Party of European Socialists, led by a British MEP, Pauline Green who gives her personal view of the Parliament below.

'The European Parliament is the only multi-national Parliament in the world, and being only 16 years old as a directly elected assembly, its role is at an early stage of evolution. Our role in my view is not to "ape" the role of national parliaments, but rather to take a fresh, innovative look at the role of this unique, multi-national Parliament which must not and does not wish to compete with national Parliaments, but rather to act in conjunction with them.

If the European Union as a concept is to work and not flounder in a morass of nationalistic, xenophobic sentiment, then the development of these relationships is crucial. Yes, the European Parliament has real influence on domestic legislation. The last piece of legislation I piloted through parliament resulted in 60% of my amendments ending up in domestic law in Britain – not bad for a MEP under a Tory government!

Yet the democratic deficit remains and the Parliament is determined to address it. The people of Europe will only have proper control of decision-making at European level when their national Parliaments control (perhaps even mandate) their national ministers going to meetings in Brussels; and the European Parliament properly controls the institutions of the Council and the Commission.

When we talk about "more powers" for the European Parliament we are referring to the re-weighting of the balance of powers within the institutions of Europe – not more powers from national Parliaments!

One thing is for sure, there are many areas of policy and legislation which only the European Parliament can impact upon. Democracy demands it be given the ability to do so.'

Pauline Green, MEP for London North and Leader of the Group of the Party of European Socialists.

The parliamentary committees

Parliament's work is prepared in 20 Committees. Each Member belongs to one or more specialist Committee, as follows:

- Foreign Affairs, Security and Defence Policies;
- Agriculture and Rural Development;
- Budgets;
- Economic and Monetary Affairs and Industrial Policy;
- Research, Technological Development and Energy;
- External Economic Relations;
- Legal Affairs and Citizens' Rights;
- Social Affairs and Employment;
- Regional Policy;
- Transport and Tourism;
- Environment, Public Health and Consumer Protection;
- Youth, Culture, Education and the Media;
- Development and Co-operation;
- Civil Liberties and Internal Affairs;
- Budgetary Control;
- Institutional Affairs;
- Fisheries;
- Rules of Procedure, the Verification of Credentials and Immunities;
- Women's Rights;
- Petitions.

The Committee of the Environment, Public Health and Consumer Protection, chaired by British MEP Ken Collins, is one of the largest of the EP's permanent committees and is probably the committee which is most relevant to the health care sector's interests. In the context of public health, the Committee has been concerned with labelling and advertising of tobacco products, pharmaceutical products, the *Europe Against Cancer* programme and food policy. It is also involved in discussions concerning the trade in human organs for transplantation purposes, the care of the terminally ill, the prevention of cardiovascular disease and the regulation of medical devices.

Ken Collins writes:
'Glancing at any newspaper across Europe, one sees articles every day relating to health, whether it be on the incidence of asthma in cities, advice on lowering cholesterol intake, statistics on cardiovascular disease, or the spread of an epidemic far away from Europe. What this demonstrates very clearly is the high level of public interest in the subject of health.

Thanks to Article 129 of the Treaty on European Union, Europe has new co-ordinating responsibilities for safeguarding our general health. Now the Union can take action to promote good health through various education campaigns as well as programmes to combat major threats such as drugs, cancer and AIDS.

The challenges that the European Union can address vary immensely, from how best to care for an ageing population to those relating to increasing population mobility, both into the Union and between Member States. Diseases arising from environmental changes and hazards in the workplace also must be addressed along with rising expectations about what health services can and should deliver. Another area involves the various issues arising from the internal market in over-the-counter pharmaceuticals and prescription medicine.

An understanding of the scale and importance of this task prompted the European Parliament into action. In June 1993, some months before the Union treaty came into force, the Parliament's Committee on the Environment, Public Health and Consumer Protection held a public hearing to examine current problems and explore policy priorities for the development of a truly European public health policy. Subsequently, the Parliament approved a report written by me and calling for three major initiatives: the creation of a European epidemiological investigation unit, an annual "State of health in Europe" report, and health promotion campaigns to be carried out in each of the Member States.

The report stressed that the European Union should bring "added value" to the work already being done nationally. Therefore, the Union should not and will not tinker with national health services: the delivery of health care is clearly better organised at the national and local levels. Instead, the Union will concentrate on activities which complement and reinforce national efforts by helping to combat major diseases and promote good health.

A vivid illustration of the way the Union can contribute is to look at rare diseases and disorders. Within the population of one Member State alone, there may be only a few cases of a specific disease in a given year. Often there may be insufficient resources or data in one Member State to provide for research into, and treatment of, such an "orphan" disease. Across Europe, however, there may be seventy or eighty such cases, thereby making research and development work at EU level more viable and appropriate.

Therefore, it would be useful to establish data networks at EU level to assist the medical professionals developing and delivering treatment, along with exchange and training programmes for professionals and also to provide more financial support for research programmes and projects, to name but a few areas for action. This is why we Members of the European Parliament welcome the Commission proposals in each of these categories.

Currently there are several important proposals, in various stages of the legislative process, being considered by the European institutions. The Committee is considering the Common positions reached on the AIDS, Cancer and Drugs programmes as well as the health promotion programme. We are also expecting a Commission Communication on health data and indicators. It is important that we arrive at common definitions on such issues as notifiable diseases, communicable diseases and even hospital beds. Such apparently minor matters can lead to severe arguments if they are not resolved at an early stage.

The European debate on health is in its infancy. Action at European level can successfully complement the activities of those responsible for health within the Member States, but at present the EU's level of legal competence in the health field is comparatively limited. The growth of European health policy and initiatives requires active political support and we in the European Parliament look to Europe's citizens and most specifically those involved in the healthcare field (and concerned enough to be reading this book!) to help us to achieve that.'

Ken Collins, MEP for Strathclyde East and Chair of the European Parliament's Committee on the Environment, Public Health and Consumer Protection.

In addition to its 20 Standing Committees, Parliament can also set up sub-committees, temporary committees and committees of enquiry, which examine more specific problems within the EU, such as drugs and racism.

When the Council requests an opinion from the Parliament, the Parliamentary Committees carry out the groundwork in preparation for Parliament's responses by appointing a member as rapporteur for each topic under consideration. The committees may also draw up a report on their own initiative, after requesting permission from the Parliament's Bureau.

Work at plenary sessions (i.e. when the Parliament meets as a whole) includes parliamentary questions, urgent debates on topical issues, statements by other institutions and voting sessions. When dealing with a piece of legislation in plenary session, Parliament votes first on the amendments, then on the draft as a whole and finally on the accompanying resolution. The latter is known as a 'legislative' resolution in cases where Parliament is consulted by the Council on a Commission proposal. Parliament's opinion is embodied in the resolution, which indicates whether it approves, rejects or amends the draft Community law.

Other institutions

The Committee of the Regions (COR)

This new committee, made up of representatives from regional and local authorities throughout the Union, was established by the Union Treaty and is intended to provide greater democratic consultation and accountability. The Committee is consulted by the Commission and the Council of Ministers on aspects of Community policy affecting the regions (including public health) and may submit independent reports on matters of specific regional interest. Interestingly, it was the subject of controversy between the UK government and local authorities, after the government had let it be known that UK representatives might be drawn from the regional Government Offices rather than being local elected representatives, or county councillors. This was seen by local authorities as a central government attempt to establish some control of the Committee, and discourage direct lines of communication to open up between local politicians and the European Commission. A 'Europe of the Regions' is not something the UK government has generally felt happy in contemplating, whilst other European countries with a strata of regional government regard this direct relationship as perfectly normal.

Councillor Roy Cross, who is a member of the Committee, comments on his experience of it to date.

'The Committee of the Regions was set up by the Treaty of Maastricht and has 223 members from all 15 states of the European Union. The United Kingdom has 24 members, all from local authorities, 14 of which are in England. The purpose of the Committee is to act as a consultative body which gives opinions, based on regional knowledge, requirements and experience, on proposals from the European Commission or the Council of Ministers.

The first plenary session was held in March 1994 and since then there have been another six (i.e. up to July 1995). To facilitate the gathering of opinions, eleven commissions and five sous-committees have been formed. These choose a rapporteur to prepare a draft opinion which is discussed and amended within the commission and then presented to the plenary session of the Committee for approval. Commission 8 and its sous-commission deal with health matters, and the subjects for opinions given so far have included the Europe Against AIDS programme, the quality of bathing water, action to prevent cancer, the effects of the use of somatropin in milk production and action to combat drugs. Each of these opinions have had a qualifying or amending effect, and publication of EU proposals so far show that in every case, the COR opinion has had an influence on the legislation produced.

There are divisive factors in the COR, however, as in all international or even national bodies. These have tended to be North versus South, highlands versus lowlands, and party political considerations, but these have not as yet caused an impasse. As members get to know one another, the work becomes more detailed and more significant.

Members do not receive a salary but claim their travelling expenses and receive a daily allowance which has recently been increased: initially it barely met the overnight hotel bill. Appointments were made for four years and so the reckoning will come in 1998!'

Cllr Roy Cross, Member of Richmondshire District Council and the Committee of the Regions.

The Economic and Social Committee (ECOSOC)

This committee, based in Brussels, represents employer and employee organizations and other interest groups. It acts in an advisory role, and must be consulted by the Council and the Commission on certain legislation. It is another mechanism for involving Europe's citizens in the decision-making process. Members are nominated by their own Member State.

The Committee now numbers 222 members, 24 from the UK. The Committee has a system of study groups, with a Chairperson and a Rapporteur. Health issues are mainly dealt with by the Social Group.

The European Court of Justice

The Court is the final arbiter in matters of Community law and overrides national law. It consists of 15 judges, one from each Member State who are chosen for six-year terms by common agreement among EU governments. The Court is assisted by six advocates general whose task is to make an analysis of each case and draw up preliminary conclusions. These do not bind the court in its final judgements. The Court has the power to settle disputes between the EU institutions: for instance, the European Parliament won a case against the Council of Ministers for failure to implement a transport policy.

Member State governments can bring actions against the EU institutions and vice versa. So if the Commission fails to persuade a Member State to implement legislation properly, it may bring the matter to the Court for judgement. A Member State which believes that the Council has decided something contrary to EU law may also bring an action against the Council.

Individuals, organizations and companies ('natural or legal persons') can appeal against EU decisions to the Court, as they frequently do in competition cases when the Commission has decided that certain behaviour is against EU rules and has perhaps even fined the company concerned. A subsidiary court, called the Court of First Instance, has been set up to deal with this type of case, with right of appeal to the European Court.

Many of the cases dealt with by the Court of Justice are referred to it by courts and tribunals within the Member States. These 'referrals' arise when a case has come before a national court involving aspects of EU law which are not entirely clear. The European Court's judgement is binding and will guide the national court in its final decision. The Court's judgements thus become part of the legal framework of every

Member State. Substantial changes have consequently been made, particularly to employment legislation, for example, in regard to rights for pregnant women. (Readers in the UK will no doubt remember the celebrated cases of young women dismissed from the armed forces on becoming pregnant, who subsequently won considerable compensatory payments after a ruling by the European Court.)

The European Court of Justice should not be confused with the European Court of Human Rights, which developed from the Council of Europe's European Convention on Human Rights and is not an institution of the European Union.

Current structures relevant to health care

The EU institutions do not interact particularly smoothly at present, due to the way in which EU involvement in the area of public health was evolved. Health Ministers of Member States meet at EU level and this is likely to occur more regularly post-Maastricht. Other key structures or groups are:

- The European Parliament: Committee on the Environment, Public Health and Consumer Protection;
- The European Commission: High level Committee of Public Health Experts (set up in 1991 and consisting of representatives of Member States meeting as an advisory committee to the Commission);
- The High Protection Advisory Committee (three specialists per Member State, chaired by the Commission).

As far as responsibility for overseeing the range of EU health programmes goes, a compromise seems to have been reached between the Commission's desire for a committee with a largely advisory function and the desire of Member States for a management committee with wider executive powers over the implementation of the health programmes. A committee is being set up to combine aspects of both functions, with representatives appointed by the Member States.

Programme/project-specific groups

Other groups have been set up on a time-limited or project-specific basis, for example, to undertake the overseeing of an awareness-raising campaign such as in the case of the European Year of Older People, or to act as a panel of experts on a particular issue. One example would be the European Committee of Cancer Experts, which acts as an advisory panel to the *Europe Against Cancer* programme. (There is also a *Europe Against AIDS* programme – more on this later.) In addition, committees of experts are brought together to assist in the drafting of EU legislation. Again, these groups meet on a time-limited basis and cease to operate when their task is complete.

European agencies

Various official agencies have been set up to act as lead bodies on specialist areas. (There have been delays in establishing some of these because of squabbling over where they should be sited).

For example:

- The European Environmental Agency (sited in Copenhagen);
- The European Monitoring Centre for Drugs and Drug Addiction (sited in Lisbon);
- The European Agency for the Evaluation of Medical Products (sited in London);
- The Agency for Health & Safety at Work (sited in Bilbao);
- The Office for Veterinary and Plant Health Inspection and Control (based in Ireland);
- The European Training Foundation (based at Turin);
- Europol and the Europol Drugs Unit (The Hague).

The European Commission also has its own research body, The European Foundation for the Improvement of Living and Working Conditions, which is based in Dublin. Much of its work is either directly or indirectly related to health and social issues, and one of its publications, *The Health Sector in the European Community: 1992 and Beyond* is a discussion document which highlights the major implications for the health sector of the Single Market and closer European union.

European Union legislation

Different types of legislation

Under the European treaties, the EU institutions may make regulations, issue directives, take decisions, make recommendations or deliver opinions.

Regulations have general application and are directly applicable in all Member States. They do not have to be confirmed by national Parliaments in order to have binding legal effect. If there is a conflict between a regulation and existing national law, the regulation overrides the national law. In fact, regulations are rarely issued and directives are more the norm as far as general legislation is concerned.

Directives are binding on Member States in terms of their objectives, which must be achieved within a stated period. Implementation is left to national governments, which interpret the directive via legislation tailored to their own circumstances and contexts. In the UK this may take the form of primary legislation, Statutory Instruments made under relevant specific powers, or an Order under the European Communities Act 1972. A directive does not have legal force in Member States on its own, but it must be translated into the law of the land within the time specified, or the Member State is liable to be penalized for not complying with it. The essential content of the directive must also be preserved and Member State governments must not dilute or distort it during its translation into national law. Directives on equality between the sexes and also on the right of female workers to take maternity leave have had a marked effect on the lives of millions of women in the EU.

Decisions are specific to particular parties and binding on those to whom they are addressed, whether Member States, companies or individuals. Decisions imposing financial obligations are also enforceable in national courts.

Recommendations and **Opinions** have no binding force but merely state the view of the institution that issues them. They may indicate strong views or intentions, however, and provide an insight into possible future legislation.

How decisions are made

The Co-operation (qualified majority voting) Procedure

This was introduced as a way of speeding up the passage of legislation on matters relating to the establishment of the Single Market. If absolute agreement on a proposal is not needed by the Council of Ministers, the new procedure allows for the adoption of a common position by a qualified majority. It is then referred for a second reading to the European Parliament. Parliament must either approve the position, adopt no position, propose amendments, or reject the position by an absolute majority (see Figure 3).

The consultation (unanimous voting) procedure

Draft proposals are prepared by the Commission, and each proposal is submitted to the Council of Ministers, which simultaneously seeks the views of the European Parliament and the Economic and Social Committee (ECOSOC). The proposals are then returned to the Commission where they may be subject to amendment and issued in a revised form for consideration by the Council of Ministers. A decision is taken to either adopt or reject each proposal.

Extended majority voting

The use of majority voting in the Council of Ministers has been extended to those aspects of environmental, health, education and consumer affairs policy which are best handled

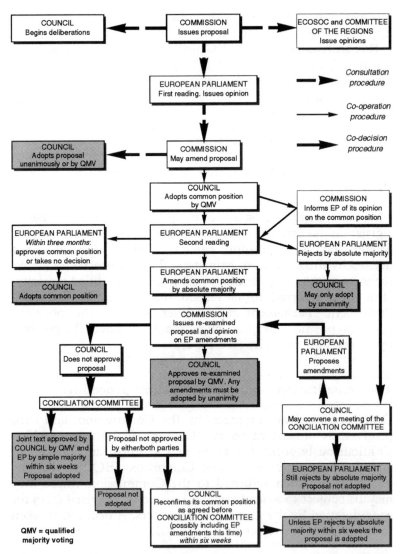

Figure 3 The decision-making process of the European Union. Reproduced with kind permission of the Local Government International Bureau's European Information Service.

on a community-wide basis. Typical areas include the promotion of student exchanges and language teaching, the fight against international environmental problems and measures to prevent the spread of disease. However, unanimous voting will still apply to those aspects of these policy areas best handled on a national basis, such as the organization of national education or health services, the choice of energy sources or measures affecting local planning procedures.

Case law

Significant cases have been brought before the European Court of Justice with regard to interpretation of EC Directives. This establishes precedents which become part of case law and often have an impact upon the everyday lives of Europe's citizens. (Many of these have focused on the issue of equal treatment of men and women and have resulted in changes to working practices and conditions.)

The importance of discussion documents and European Union White Papers

These are documents which are indications of the way in which policy is developing and in the case of White Papers, the forerunners of new legislation.

The most important are:

- Commission Proposals;
- European Parliament Reports;
- Opinions and Reports of the Economic and Social Committee.

The European Commission issues Green Papers from time to time which seek to stimulate wide-ranging discussion about future action at Union level before any concrete proposals emerge. Unfortunately, in the UK, and in the field of health care generally, few respond to these important and influential discussion documents. For example, the Green Paper entitled

Social Policy – Options for the Union invited responses from concerned organizations, professionals and citizens but few UK-based health and social care organizations participated in the debate. (The White Paper which followed, *European Social Policy – A Way Forward for the Union* is discussed in a later chapter.)

Copies of the papers can be obtained directly from Brussels as well as from the official source in the UK (HMSO) and there is usually a reasonable period of time in which to respond.

The Maastricht Treaty

The Maastricht Treaty builds on the achievements of the European Community, paving the way for 'ever closer union', both economically and politically, including the introduction of a single currency. The next logical step is a completely frontier-free market and the establishment of new political structures to enable the Community to fulfil its responsibilities as a leading global power in a rapidly changing world.

The Treaty was based upon two inter-governmental conferences, one on Economic and Monetary Union and the other on Political Union, both running in parallel. Inter-governmental conferences (IGCs) are the usual way of agreeing new European treaties or changing existing ones.

The final text of the Union Treaty changed existing Articles of the Treaty of Rome and added extra ones, and new protocols were agreed for certain new policy areas. In preparation for the work to be done on Economic and Monetary Union (EMU), a Committee was set up consisting of the governors of the national central banks (like the Bank of England) and independent experts, and subsequent negotiations were based on their advice.

The Union Treaty's scope is wider than that of previous treaties and it opens up new policy areas and extends the responsibilities of the European institutions. One important new concept introduced is that of **European Union citizenship**. This is not a vague, abstract ideal, but exists as a concrete set of rights and entitlements including:

- the right to reside in another Member State;
- the right to vote and stand as a candidate in local and European elections in other Member States;
- the right to diplomatic or consular protection by any European Member State (i.e. if you are in a country where your own state has no diplomatic representation, you can seek assistance at any EU Member State embassy);
- the right to petition the European Parliament.

The Union Treaty also extended the **powers of the European Parliament** (as already indicated in the section on the EP). The European Parliament still does not have the powers of a national parliament but it does now have some powers of joint decision-making with the Council of Ministers. It can also request the Commission to make proposals for new legislation if this is deemed necessary, and can set up Committees of Enquiry if it has reason to believe any maladministration or corruption has occurred. If citizens petition the Parliament, a special ombudsman appointed by the EP will deal with their grievances.

The Treaty also tightened up **financial and budgetary controls**, and gave the Parliament a role in that it can require evidence from the Commission of proper financial management and accounting.

Two separate pillars within the Treaty are common policies on **foreign and security matters** and **justice and home affairs**. Both are controversial and difficult areas. In the case of the first pillar, the new provisions allow for Member States to act as a Union in matters of foreign policy and to take action which would be binding on member countries. Defence policy is further complicated by the fact that some EU Member States are members of the Western European Union (WEU – based in London but moving to Brussels – and others are members of NATO (the North Atlantic Treaty Organization). The Union Treaty states that national defence policies must not be prejudiced, NATO obligations must be respected but the WEU will be developed as the defence component of the EU. The defence provisions are to be revised in 1998 and defence and foreign policy is likely to be a major theme in the 1996 IGC.

In terms of justice and home affairs, areas of common interest include asylum policy, immigration, and co-operation between police and customs on crime and smuggling.

The 'free movement' principles enshrined in the Single European Act have yet to be fully implemented, with the most controversial being the free movement of people and the elimination of customs barriers to enable this. A number of EU countries (including France, Germany and Belgium) formed a 'Union within a Union' when they undertook to abolish internal borders – an agreement made at Schengen and named accordingly – but the UK has always been determined to maintain its border checks and remains outside the Schengen Group.

The section of the Treaty dealing with new **social policy** matters was taken out of the main body of the document because the UK government refused to sign the Treaty with it in. It therefore became the subject of a Protocol agreement, whereby the other Member States committed themselves to progress the measures identified under the 'Social Charter'. Wherever possible, the Council of Ministers will try to gain agreement from all Member States on items of social legislation, but if the UK government is in disagreement, the other States will go ahead without them. Legislation agreed in these circumstances would not be binding in the UK. This is known as 'the UK opt-out'. With regard to health care, the most obvious addition and area of greatest potential impact is the public health article. **Article 129 (The Public Health Article)** gives a degree of legal competence in the area of public health to the European Commission, which enables it to draft legislation on the issues involved. (For the wording of the Public Health Article and an account of its significance, refer to Chapter 4.)

The Treaty also aims to increase consumer choice, improve the protection of the environment, create employment opportunities and award new rights to the citizens of Europe. However, there is concern from a number of influential players on the EU scene that the Chapter does not go far enough and that the competence of the European institutions in relation to health matters should be increased.

European decision-making and the policy of openness

The European Commission has stated that it is committed to a greater degree of openness in European decision-making and provision of information, and this is supported by the European Parliament. However, this has not been matched by a commitment from the Council of Ministers, which is actually the most powerful of all the European institutions. Although the Council had agreed a code of conduct promising the 'widest possible access' to documents, requests from journalists and others for certain minutes and other papers were routinely denied on the grounds of protecting the interests of the institution and the confidentiality of its proceedings.

In October 1995, the European Court ruled that documents had been unlawfully denied to a *Guardian* journalist, John Carvel, by the Council of Ministers. *The Guardian* had been supported in its campaign by the European Parliament and the governments of Denmark and the Netherlands, as strong supporters of openness.

John Carvel subsequently wrote in *The Guardian*, that, following his posting to Brussels, he had come to the conclusion that the Council of Ministers 'operated under rules that were alien to the European democratic tradition'. The citizens of Europe were being subjected to laws created by the Council, without being allowed to know what was being done in their name.

'In London the Eurosceptics tended to rave against the European Commission as if it were to blame for everything which diminished national sovereignty. They got it wrong. The Commission's job has always been to propose new laws and administer existing ones. The real power to decide whether legislation passes – and in what form – lay with the ministers of member states, subject to a little tinkering at the margins by the MEPs.' (*The Guardian*, 1995.)

The decision was all the more important because it was brought as an action by a private citizen. Greater openness of Council proceedings is now likely to become an issue for the 1996 Inter-governmental Conference.

The European Union and the British press

Almost every newspaper story on the European Union which appears in the British press is either written from a negative or critical perspective (such as many of the items on fishing rights or subsidies for agriculture) or from a basis of inaccuracy and misrepresentation. Perhaps British editors believe that these attitudes sell papers, and that the accuracy of an item is unimportant. Stories about the bent banana, the proposed suppression of saucy seaside postcards and the standardization of condoms have all appeared in the press and been given some credence, when they were all unfounded. 'Tales of "barmy" European law are meat and drink to the headline writers. These stories are often pure fiction, or garbled accounts of perfectly sensible measures. They do real damage because they play on popular fears and prejudices.' (The Right Honourable Malcolm Rifkind MP in *Do you* still *believe all you read in the newspapers?* published by the European Commission in the UK.)

More importantly, in their quest to report on the apparently bizarre and bureaucratic world of the 'Eurocrats' in Brussels, most British newspapers have consistently omitted to report on major policy initiatives and developments.

Summary points

1 Political control over the Union rests firmly with the leaders and ministers of the Member States.
2 The Commission does not have the size, power or pretensions to rival the governments of Member States, let alone become a Euro-State.
3 The relatively late arrival of health on the European agenda has been a handicap. It does not have a separate directorate devoted to it, so that health practitioners have to find their way around a complicated maze.
4 The increase in the 'power of Brussels' is really a re-weighting of the balance of interests, to redress the democratic deficit. The enlargement of the scope of the European Parliament and its committee system, the

Committee of the Regions and the Economic and Social Committee might seem at first glance to offer a bureaucrats' charter. In reality they are an attempt to give a more direct form of participation in European affairs to citizens and interest groups within the Member States.

5 In health, as in other matters, the professed function of the Union is not to duplicate or take over the role of the Member States and their internal agencies, but to take supplementary and complementary action and do those things which can be most effective at international level.

6 European law has not usurped national law. It has been adopted as part of the legal framework of each Member State.

7 Decision-making in the Union takes a variety of forms which are sensitive to national interests. Legislation is usually preceded by discussion documents and Green Papers. The opportunity for debate and influence has been under-utilized so far by UK health care interests.

8 The Maastricht Treaty was an ambitious and controversial step forward, laying a foundation for ever closer union, with monetary and political connotations. At a more prosaic level, it has extended the powers of the European Parliament, given some concrete meaning to European citizenship, and introduced a Social Chapter – subject to a UK opt-out. The Public Health Article (Article 129) of the treaty gives the Commission some legal competence in the field of public health for the first time, but critics claim that it does not go far enough.

References and further reading

Carvel, J. (1995). *The Guardian*, 20 October.
The European. (1992). Maastricht Made Simple.

4

European health and social policy

Aims of this Chapter

In this chapter, we aim to:
- explain the rationale for a social dimension at EU level;
- outline the relationship between European economic and social policy;
- explain the legal basis for social legislation, and specifically health;
- outline the development of the social dimension;
- describe in brief the aims and objectives of the EU's social policy;
- focus in some detail on the EU's policy in relation to health;
- summarize the EU Framework document for action in the field of public health.

The European Union is now the most exciting laboratory for international co-operation in the world.

The Right Honourable Paddy Ashdown MP.
The Walter Sicket Memorial lecture, April 1995.

The social dimension of the European Union

Although economic aims have been the strongest driving forces towards European union, there has also been a social movement, which is now gaining momentum. This has been a controversial development, frequently beset by problems and lack of agreement between members. Some Member State governments, including the UK, would have preferred to have concentrated almost entirely on market issues and to have limited any social legislation to matters concerned with health and safety at work and employment issues. The majority of EU states did not agree, and there was a backbone of commitment to a social dimension for the Union within the European Commission. The Commission's former President, Jacques Delors, was firm in his conviction that economic union could not be properly and fairly achieved without social union. The four freedoms, after all, included freedom of movement for people (as well as goods, services and capital).

In common with the rest of the industrialized world, Europe is now experiencing profound changes, and social policy at European level is seen as playing a vital part in meeting the resultant challenge. The Commission's view, frequently articulated, is that the Union's economic strength and prosperity in the world arena will depend on its capacity to build an active, open and fair society, which can mobilize the energies and talents of its people and improve their quality of life, both as workers and citizens. The counter-argument is that European social legislation hampers competitiveness and economic buoyancy and does not take account of local conditions. This case has been put most frequently and forcibly by the British government, which believes that social legislation should largely be the domain of national governments. The social dimension is clearly quite broad in scope and covers areas relating to people, both as workers and as citizens.

The Social Charter and the later Social Chapter are only a part of this dimension, as they deal primarily with *employment-related* issues. As already explained, the UK government is the only signatory of the Union Treaty to refuse to accept the Social Chapter – a Chapter therefore taken out of the Treaty and incorporated into a separate Protocol.

The 'Social Charter'

Predating the Union Treaty was the 'Social Charter' – a document committing Member States to a series of social policy objectives as part of the Single Market completion programme. Its full title was the 'Community Charter of Basic Social Rights of Workers', and it was drafted by the Commission in May 1989 and considerably watered down in the resultant debate. Despite the dilution, the UK refused to sign it at the Strasbourg Summit in December 1989, but it was adopted by the other 11 Member States despite British dissent. It was not a law but a 'solemn declaration' which bound the signatories to upholding the social rights it described. The Social Charter set out a range of basic employment rights under 12 headings:

- free movement of workers within the EC (as it was then);
- 'fair remuneration' for employment;
- improvement and approximation of conditions of employment;
- social security;
- freedom of association and collective bargaining;
- vocational training;
- equal treatment for men and women;
- information, consultation and participation arrangements;
- health and safety in the workplace;
- young people;
- retired people;
- disabled people.

The Charter was actually no more than a statement of commitment to specified principles. However, the rights outlined within it were then expressed within an Action Programme intended to implement the Charter, and used as a framework for the Commission's initiatives (including draft legislation) within the social sphere from 1990 to 1993. Fifty measures were identified, some of which were proposed as legally binding Directives but others were simply put forward as recommendations to the Member States. The whole Charter was pursued as an area for the subsidiarity principle, with the introduction to the Action Programme making this fully explicit:

> In accordance with the principle of subsidiarity whereby the Community acts when the set objectives can be reached more effectively at its level than at that of the Member States. . . . The Commission takes the view that responsibility for the initiatives to be taken as regards the implementation of social rights lies with the Member States, their constituent parts or the two sides of industry as well as, within the limits of its powers, with the European Community.
>
> Social Charter Action Program. 1989

(In other words, intervention will only take place at European level if the objective fails to be achieved by the Member States.)

Many of the measures identified under the Social Charter Action Programme made very slow progress. Some were becalmed for lengthy periods when no agreement could be reached on them. Others were so diluted that they became irrelevant to Member States which already had more stringent social protection legislation in place (for example, in the case of employment protection legislation for pregnant women and maternity leave).

Margaret Thatcher's government was implacably opposed to the Social Charter and its implications. In the post-Thatcher era, this attitude softened, but only slightly. The subsequent government of John Major was still opposed to the Charter and its principles and indeed to anything which it perceived as over-regulation of the labour market. The UK government was also annoyed at the way that some directives had been put forward, in the sense of the decision-making procedure utilized. The Single European Act (1986) had incorporated a new Article on health and safety of workers (Article 118a) and any legislation proposed under this Article could be agreed by qualified majority voting, because it was part of the 'Single Market programme'. This kind of voting procedure was obviously more likely to result in agreement than unanimous voting. Some of the Social Charter legislation was put forward under this basis, including the directive on protection of pregnant workers, and the British government objected to the Treaty base, seeing it as a sneaky move to get the legislation through.

The Social Chapter

With the next stage in the process of European union, the Maastricht Treaty, an attempt was made to update and extend articles relating to social policy and provide a new legal basis for action. In other words, to translate the good intentions expressed in the Social Charter into a Chapter of the Maastricht Treaty covering social policy. But the UK was again unwilling to accept its provisions; undeterred, the other 11 Member States signed up to a separate protocol agreement, outside the Treaty – the Social Chapter or Social Protocol.

The main aims of the Social Chapter are to improve living and working conditions, promote employment, encourage dialogue between the two sides of industry and ensure social protection. For countries which are signatories, the following matters can be dealt with by **qualified** majority voting:

- health and safety;
- working conditions;
- workers' information and consultation;
- equality at work between men and women.

Unanimous voting is required in the areas of:

- social security and social protection of workers;
- protection for workers made redundant;
- representation and collective defence of workers' and employers' interests;
- conditions of employment for non-EU nationals.

(NB The Protocol does not cover pay, the right of association, nor the right to strike or take similar industrial action.) The Protocol provides the opportunity for management and workers – the 'Social Partners' – to submit proposals in these areas. The 'two sides of industry' are perceived by the Commission as being important players on the European policy front, and this view of them as social partners is indicative of an attitude which prevails in other parts of the European Union, in contrast to the UK tendency to perceive them as natural opponents. This fundamental difference in perception is at the root of certain disagreements between the UK and other Member States, although it would be naive to assume that this is the sole reason for policy divergence between the UK and its partner nations or the European institutions.

Nonetheless, the Maastricht Treaty itself extended the scope of previous treaties by opening up new social policy fields, like education and health, as well as granting new powers to the European Parliament. It places more emphasis on member states working together and closer co-operation, in order to bring about improvements and raise standards. It also attempts to involve European citizens far more than ever before in the decision-making processes. Article 2 of the Union Treaty sums up the social goals identified:

to promote throughout the Community a harmonious and balanced development of economic activities, sustainable and non-inflationary growth respecting the environment, a high degree of convergence of economic performance, a high level of employment and social protection, the raising of the standard of living and quality of life, and economic and social cohesion and solidarity among Member States.

Treaty of European Union. 1992

Options for the Union

In 1993, the Commissioner for Social Affairs and Employment, Padraig Flynn, issued his Green Paper on European Social Policy. *Options for the Union*, as it was called, was intended to encourage wide-ranging debate about the future direction of social policy. It began by asking the question: 'What sort of a society do Europeans want?', and invited responses from EU institutions, Member States, employers, trade unions, organizations and ordinary citizens. It summarized the challenges and changes affecting European societies as:

- the globalization of trade and production;
- the impact of new technologies on work, society and individuals;
- the ageing of the population;
- persistently high levels of unemployment.

The Green Paper focused on these problems and others, and suggested some ways forward, with questions on how the European Union should tackle each area. Unsurprisingly, those who responded were mainly from organizations and institutions, particularly special interest groups. Even though the Green Paper was issued free, in a glossy cover with numerous colour photographs and illustrations, its circulation was fairly narrow. Most students and members of the public were unaware of any consultation, largely because it went unnoticed and unreported by the press and mass media generally, to whom it was a 'non-story'.

The Social Policy White Paper

From the debate on the Green Paper there followed a White Paper, *European Social Policy – A Way Forward for the Union*. This set out the framework or main lines of action at Union level for the coming years, and sought to stimulate increased collaboration between governments, social partners and civic and voluntary organizations. It was based on the principle that Europe needs a broadly-based, innovative and forward-looking social policy. Job creation will be at the top of the agenda for the period 1995–99, but social policy goes beyond employment. It affects people both inside and outside work – their family life, their health and their old age – and is essentially about the quality of life.

The measures outlined in the White Paper aimed to consolidate and build on the European Community's past achievements, particularly in relation to employment law, health and safety, free movement of people and equal treatment of men and women. Going further than this, they aimed to create a 'new dynamic' by producing proposals to strengthen these improvements and take action in additional areas, such as social protection, equal opportunities for all (not just between the sexes) and public health.

A number of fundamental questions central to the development of European social policy were also raised in the Commission's White Paper on *Growth, Competitiveness and Employment*, presented by Jacques Delors at the European Council meeting in Brussels in December 1993. This concluded that competitiveness was crucial for wealth and job creation and that there needed to be a re-orientation in this direction in European labour market policies. These principles were used to inform the policy measures outlined in the Social Policy White Paper. The social measures focused around some 'guiding principles' for the future role of the Union, as follows.

Social and economic integration: employment is the key

The highest priority should be given to the creation of new jobs and to integrating people into society. This is seen as the only way of financing social policy systems.

Competitiveness and social progress: two sides of the same coin

Europe needs to compete in world markets and develop an efficient, quality-based economy with significant investment in new technologies. The key resource in this is a well-educated, adaptable and highly motivated population.

Convergence which respects diversity

The European Union's diverse cultures are part of its richness. Total harmonization is not the goal, but rather a converging of common objectives so that we can progress in harmony, rather than force uniformity on different countries which have different perceptions and needs.

A level playing field of common minimum standards

These standards should not over-stretch the economically weaker Member States but neither should they hold back the more developed. Low social standards should not be used to create a 'cheap labour' society which would result in unfair economic competition. The aim should be to improve standards across all Member States.

Achievement of these goals was envisaged via a number of means, including legislation, collective agreements, financial incentives and support, encouragement of co-operation between Member States, better information which is more widely available and analysis of future trends.

Throughout the whole of the White Paper, there is an underlying emphasis on education and training. The key to prosperity is seen as a well-educated workforce, able to acquire new skills and retrain as necessary, which is adaptable and motivated. 'Social exclusion', that is, the exclusion of certain groups of people from the labour market and from other benefits in society (i.e. access to good housing, education, and health) is identified as a negative and damaging factor and every effort should be made to ensure social integration of all groups in society. Underpinning these is the need for effective health promotion, because the link between health and economic and social prosperity is unarguable.

(Note: the White Paper goes into much more detail on these issues and is well worth reading, despite being written in 'Euro-speak' and riddled with jargon and technical phrases. If readers become impatient with this style, it is worth remembering that every document of this kind has to be translated rapidly and may not have been drafted originally in English.)

Health at the forefront of social policy

The legal basis for a European Union health policy now exists as part of the Maastricht Treaty. Before that, European health policy (indeed all European policies) had its origins in the early days of the EU when it was related to 'Common Market' issues. But even within this limited context, the actions of the EU have from the outset taken account of the need to protect human health. Chapter III of the Treaty of Rome (1957) was devoted to health and safety, and the standards set then to protect the health of workers have been revised several times. In the 1986 Single European Act, the provision most related to health is Article 100a, paragraph 3, which states that when the Commission engages in harmonization measures, those measures must be based on a 'high level of health protection'. Additionally, Article 118a of the SEA, addressing health and safety at work, gave further impetus to Community competence in the field of health, albeit in a narrow context. The progress made towards realizing the Single Market aims of free movement of people, goods and services have also had an impact on a range of health-related matters such as pharmaceuticals.

Looking back at previous Community policies and instruments of direct relevance to health protection, there has clearly been positive action taking place, despite the absence of a strong legal basis. Links between public health and other areas such as environment have also been influential in assisting progress on the health front. The efforts of the European Community 'to preserve, protect and improve the quality of the environment', are at one with its responsibility 'to contribute towards protecting human health'. However, despite the lack of a strong legal basis for action, the Community's public health activities went beyond control and protection from environmental and workplace hazards to the encouragement and co-ordination of measures to combat major diseases and positively to promote health. The *Europe against Cancer* programme, 1987–89, was the first major disease prevention programme. There have been further related programmes in the period 1990–94 and a new programme is currently underway. These programmes have brought about action on smoking in public places (though legislation has not always been rigorously implemented), and on tobacco advertising and labelling. Other programmes soon followed as political pressure and health developments demanded Community action, including *Europe Against AIDS* and a European plan to combat the abuse of drugs. (See Chapter 7 for more detail on European programmes.)

Although legislation itself has brought about changes in the field of health, more informal processes also play a part. Over recent years, there has been a steady increase in pan-European organizations being set up to focus Community-wide attention on public health issues, such as the Hospital Committee of the European Community (HCEC), which together with the recently formed European Public Health Alliance (EPHA: see the case study in Chapter 8) and the Association of Schools of Public Health in the European Region (ASPHER), has been instrumental in placing health squarely on the Community agenda. Other EU institutions such as the European Parliament, the Economic and Social Committee and the Council, have each in their own way been pushing forward the European health debate for some time.

Article 129 – just the beginning?

Article 129 of the Union Treaty gives a degree of legal competence in the area of public health to the European Commission. The Article focuses on the need for co-ordination of existing national policies (as opposed to suggesting any new legislation), in order to achieve a high level of human health protection across the Union. It states that:

1 The Community shall contribute towards ensuring a high level of human health protection by encouraging co-operation between the Member States and, if necessary, lending support to their action. Community action shall be directed towards the prevention of diseases, in particular the

major health scourges, including drug dependence, by promoting research into their causes and their transmissions, as well as health information and education.

Health protection requirements shall form a constituent part of the Community's other policies.

2 Member States shall in liaison with the Commission, coordinate among themselves their policies and programmes in the areas referred to in paragraph 1. The Commission may, in close contact with the Member States, take any useful initiative to promote such co-ordination.

3 The Community and the Member States shall foster cooperation with third countries and the competent international organisations in the sphere of public health.

4 In order to contribute to the achievement of the objectives referred to in this Article, the Council: acting in accordance with the procedure referred to in Article 189b, after consulting the Economic and Social Committee and the Committee of the Regions, shall adopt incentive measures, excluding any harmonisation of the laws and regulations of the Member States; acting by a qualified majority on a proposal from the Commission, shall adopt recommendations.

Treaty of European Union. 1992

This is a very limited degree of competence and many pro-Europeans may feel it is little more than a well-meaning gesture without any genuine clout. Those who view it more positively, however, see it as a beginning, a foundation for more extended and ambitious treatment. The Maastricht Treaty is to be reviewed at the inter-governmental conference starting in 1996, and preparations have been long underway for that IGC.

Amongst other planned proposals, the European Parliament's Committee on the Environment, Public Health and Consumer Protection has approved amendments to Article 129. These were proposed by David Bowe, MEP for Cleveland and Richmond, and they could ultimately be incorporated into a report being produced by the Parliament's Institutional Affairs Committee on changes to the Maastricht Treaty. The amendments are as follows:

Paragraph 1   Community policy on Health shall contribute to the pursuit of the following objectives:

promoting health
improving health protection
promoting measures at international level to deal with regional or world-wide health problems.

Paragraph 2   Community policy on health shall aim at a high level of protection taking into account the diversity of health systems and practices in the Member States.

Paragraph 3   In preparing its policy on health, the Community shall take account of:

– age structures and disease patterns of the peoples of the Community
– increasing population mobility
– changes in the physical and work environments
– socio-economic conditions
– advances in research and technology

Paragraph 4   Health requirements must be integrated into the definition and implementation of other Community policies.

Treaty of European Union. 1992

Again, the use of phrases like 'contribute to' and 'take account of' means that there is no hint of a move towards a direct role in health care for EU institutions, even one such as monitoring of quality of health care delivery. The approach is based very much upon subsidiarity and complementarity to Member State governments, but the scope of future policy is at the same time being made more explicit, with health issues being firmly set within a global socio-economic context. This is not surprising: the European Parliament has been in favour of a Community health policy since the early 1980s and has put forward several resolutions in the field of health including the European Charter of Rights of Hospital Patients (Document 1–970/83), and Women in Childbirth (Document AZ–38/88).

The Parliament has often raised questions on the subject of health and through the various committees, in particular the Committee on Environment, Public Health, and Consumer Protection, has prepared several reports on health-related subjects including AIDS, health education, drug abuse and organ transplantation. The Economic and Social Committee has also regularly given its opinions on health matters such as dangerous substances, prevention of asbestos pollution and occupational cancer. It was on the basis of such expressions from the European institutions, together with support from numerous health professionals, medical and patient associations and interest groups, that the Treaty on European Union gave the European Commission competence to act in the field of public health, as spelt out in Article 129.

The European Commission's framework for action in the field of public health

In November 1993 the Commission put forward its framework for action in the field of public health (COM Doc (93)559) as the first tangible result of the Public Health Article. This Communication, a statement from the Commission which contains no formal proposal, did four things. It:

1 set out the major health issues confronting the European Union;
2 explained how priorities might be established;
3 described what actions were possible, and how these were related to past actions by the European Commission and Member States, and to other policies;
4 suggested a number of specific programmes.

The thrust of the framework was towards health promotion and encouragement of healthy lifestyles, in addition to accident and disease prevention. It is essentially a holistic approach to health, viewed not just in terms of the individual but within a socio-economic context. The Commission intended to discharge its new responsibility by encouraging co-operation between the Member States, with the relevant international organizations, and to support actions in the following areas which had been singled out for possible future Union action:

- health promotion, education and training;
- collecting health data and indicators, as well as monitoring and surveillance of diseases;
- cancer treatment;
- drugs;
- AIDS and other communicable diseases;
- accidents and injuries;
- pollution and related diseases;
- rare diseases.

The Communication also stresses that preventative action must not merely concentrate on particular diseases, but on the underlying causes of ill-health, not least the effects of poverty and related problems. Resources should be concentrated on reducing the impact of causal factors relating to several diseases, or to ill-health in general.

The types of action envisaged by the Communication are limited both by the likely size of available resources and the cautious terms in which the competence of the Community is defined. Of central importance will be actions in support of those undertaken by the Member States, as well as assistance in co-ordination of those actions. This will include large-scale cost-effectiveness analyses of existing and proposed measures, the formulation of proposals for new measures, and the establishment of networks designed to facilitate communication between researchers or practitioners in different Member States and beyond.

In discussing the Framework, the Commissioner for Social Affairs, Padraig Flynn, stated that 'many diseases and disorders of today are related to lifestyle factors and changes in behaviour and attitudes in areas such as diet, nutrition, exercise, smoking, alcohol abuse and hygiene could help combat their onset'. This would, he said, 'not only improve the quality of life for individuals, their families and society as a whole but would reduce pressure on health care and treatment facilities and reduce pressure on health spending in Member States'.

The Framework for Action - a Summary

The wide cultural, social and economic diversity of the Union means that Member States are confronted with a variety of health protection problems. Nonetheless, there are several common issues which confront all Member States and their respective Health Ministers:

- **an ageing population** – in 1980, about 17.5 per cent of the population was over 60 years old, but this figure may increase to about 24 per cent by the year 2010. This means that there will be more old people, who are heavy users of health services, and the burden of financing services will fall on a relatively smaller working population.
- **increasing population mobility** – migration into the Union, the coming into effect of the single market, and the general increase in travel and tourism are leading to an ever-larger intermingling of populations. This can lead to a more rapid spread of communicable diseases, increased potential for drug abuse and real difficulties in providing for the specific needs of migrant communities.
- **increases in some diseases related to environmental changes and the workplace,** including respiratory diseases and some cancers. Also on the increase are conditions relating to stress, musculoskeletal problems and conditions linked with the use of computers and other modern work-related equipment.
- **rising expectations concerning health** – growing demands on health services are accompanied by rising expectations of what these services can provide. New technologies and treatments, improved drugs and medicines are costly, and difficult choices must be made on the location of facilities and provision of services and products.
- **socio-economic problems**, in particular, social exclusion, are increasing because of slow economic growth and growing unemployment. Social exclusion, unemployment, inequalities and poverty are leading to health problems for those affected.
- **cost containment** is a major concern for all Member States and has resulted in controls on prescription of drugs and medical recruitment, together with the imposition of charges.
- **pressures on health services are likely to intensify** and lower spending would have disproportionately adverse effects on vulnerable members of society like the poor, elderly and chronically sick.
- **ensuring that EU citizens have a high standard of health is a legal and ethical obligation** placed on Member States by the Union Treaty and by the previous Council resolution of 11 November 1991.
- **the benefits of improved health protection** include avoidance of premature deaths, disablement, chronic illness and absenteeism, together with improvements in productivity and enhancement of quality of life.

Current health trends in the Member States

Lower levels of mortality, including infant mortality, is the trend in all European states. Average European life expectancy for men was 72.8 in 1989, compared with 67.3 in 1960. For women the figures were 79.2 and 72.7 respectively. Infant mortality was 34.8 per 1000 in 1960 and 8.2 in 1989. The causes of death changed significantly as a result of improved hygiene and vaccination programmes, with communicable diseases (excluding AIDS) considerably reduced. The most common causes of death are now cancer and cardiovascular diseases, with the latter beginning to decrease, and other causes, like Alzheimer's disease, on the increase.

Morbidity rates are less easy to compare because the Member States do not collect data consistently. (Morbidity rates relate to numbers of people suffering from illnesses or medical conditions.) Conditions which result in high morbidity, and also mortality rates are:

- road accidents
- cardiovascular diseases
- mental illness (including suicide)
- cancer
- musculoskeletal conditions
- respiratory diseases including asthma.

Drug dependence is also a contributory factor and is linked to various health and social problems. (Health concerns in the EU are considered in more detail in Chapter 4, Public Health: the Challenges for Europe.)

Community action and activities

Subsidiarity is the key word here: only where action is best taken at European level will there be EU legislation. The Treaty basis (i.e., Articles 3(o) and 129) focuses on preventative action and health promotion, and this is the intention of the Commission in the action programme following on from the Framework document.

The criteria for identifying diseases or conditions suitable for action at European level are as follows:

- diseases causing premature death or linked with high death rates
- diseases causing, or with the potential to cause, high morbidity or serious disability
- diseases which have a detrimental effect on quality of life and also a socio-economic effect such as high absenteeism, high treatment costs, unfitness for work

- diseases which are preventable in practical ways
- diseases which would be better tackled at European level, in terms of 'added value'.

Prime candidates under these criteria are:

Cancer is in some cases linked clearly with lifestyle.

Cardiovascular disease is already decreasing as a result of reductions in smoking and other lifestyle-related factors.

Accidents: road accidents are the leading cause of death for young people. Incidents have fallen in most Member States recently, but risen in Spain and Portugal.

Suicides have increased across Europe with the exception of Germany, though no satisfactory explanation has yet been made.

AIDS and communicable diseases: cases of AIDS and related conditions continue to increase across all member States, but the highest rates are in France, Spain and Italy, which together account for 71 per cent of all cases. Tuberculosis is also increasing.

Other diseases: mental illness, respiratory problems and musculo-skeletal conditions are linked not only with environment and stress of various kinds but with increasing age. As the population ages, this is likely to continue.

Drug dependence and **rare diseases** also rate a mention in the Framework document.

The Framework document places much emphasis on consultation with Member State governments and experts, and on promoting exchanges of experience and knowledge. Research is an area where financial incentives can encourage pan-European activity to examine the causes of ill-health across national boundaries. Current EU research includes work on prevention of illness, health care and health systems, major health problems and diseases with a socio-economic impact, medical ethics and human genome analysis. (Note: more information on EU Research programmes is provided in Chapter 7.)

The approach of the EU will be a combination of general measures such as health information, data and surveillance, and measures focusing on specific diseases and conditions, such as the *Europe Against Cancer* programme.

The following priorities for European Union action are identified:

- health promotion, education and training;
- collection of health data and indicators, and disease monitoring and surveillance;
- action against cancer;
- action against drug use and dependence (i.e. illegal substances);
- action against AIDS and communicable diseases;
- reductions in accidents and injuries;

- tackling pollution-related diseases;
- work on rare diseases.

Programmes on other health threats might be introduced in the future if necessary.

Annexes to the framework covered the preventative policies of the individual Member States and an overview of the Community policies and legal instruments relevant to health, such as health and the environment, health and safety at work, food safety, pharmaceuticals, consumer protection, medical devices, research and information technology, social security co-ordination, mutual recognition of professional qualifications and disease prevention and health promotion. A further Annexe outlined the health protection requirements within other Community policies (such as agriculture).

The Commission is conscious of the need to tread warily as far as health care is concerned, because its funding and delivery are primarily matters for the Member States. However, like education, it is one of the fundamental building blocks of a well-functioning and successful society. In addition, the creation of the EU with its 'four freedoms', especially freedom of movement of people, actually increases the potential risks and challenges in terms of health factors (these will be discussed in more detail in Chapter 6), and many other European policies have health implications. The Commission's 1995 Workplan included a new initiative on health data and indicators. DGV is also engaged in a five-year programme on pollution-related diseases (including asthma and allergies), accidents and injuries and rare diseases.

Some other general policy areas

Professional mobility

The Commission envisages that the free movement of health professionals facilitated by the Qualifications Directives (see Chapter 6), will be an important dimension in the development of a Union programme on public health.

Training programmes and exchange visits for health professionals will be an important aspect in effective health promotion and disease prevention. Increasing awareness of diseases and health problems on a European-wide basis is essential, since growing migration and travel are also encouraging the migration of certain diseases across Member States' borders. It is important to develop the training of health professionals on health promotion and disease prevention so that they are better equipped to deliver this message in their professional capacity.

European citizenship

As already stated, the Maastricht Treaty enshrines the principle that the citizens of all European Union Member States are also citizens of the Union, with the right to travel freely, work and live throughout its territory. However, the theme of European citizenship is not new, and as far back as 1973 the Copenhagen European Summit talked of a 'European Identity'. Another initiative already adopted is the 12-point European citizenship programme, which ranges from greater democracy and social legislation to a formal commitment to equality for all citizens of the Union.

Much attention has been focused on the citizen in his/her role as consumer, especially in the areas of consumer protection and safety. In theory, about 370 million European citizens are now able to choose from the broadest range of goods and services available anywhere in the world. (In practice, anomalies continue to exist like the variation in electrical plugs, television systems and cars which have to be specially manufactured for driving on the left in the UK. As people move around more freely, even only as tourists, these inconsistencies are likely to irritate and pressure will mount for them to be phased out.)

The European Commission aims to foster the emergence of a new type of consumer behaviour, more demanding and yet more responsible. The growing number of consumer interest groups and pressure groups is an indication that the public is becoming more aware of the power of the consumer and also more educated about the policy-making process, and is keen to participate. For 'Europhiles' on both sides, the compelling vision is of a Europe without internal frontiers, which allows for the continual springboarding of ideas, networking and cross-fertilization. It also requires contact with, and access to, best concepts and practice in a number of social policy areas. This approach to a dynamic citizens' Europe should also apply to the achievement of better services, better health protection and welfare, better consumer protection and a better environment in which to live and work.

Information provision and openness

One of the Commission's broadest aims is to ensure that information flows freely across the Member States, in order to enable people to understand policies and programmes, to benefit from examples of good practice and to disseminate the outcomes of developmental work. In practice, this is an expensive and difficult aim to address, both at the level of the citizen and the professional. Certainly in the case of health care data, the difficulties in collecting information on national systems and statistics are such that little useful information is accessible. A report jointly issued by the Hospital Committee of the EU (HOPE) and the International Hospital Federation in 1995 provided a critical analysis of the difficulties in collecting national information and called for the establishment of a European Observatory on health care data.

Conclusions

As the European Union itself has evolved from its narrow origins as an area of free trade, so have its policies evolved and developed to serve its population as a whole, and not simply those involved in economic activity.

The development of a 'Social Europe' has not been easy and even now is not firmly established. The refusal of the UK to allow the integration of social legislation via the Union treaty inevitably weakened the thrust of policy implementation and created a precedent of disunity. As the European Union becomes larger the problems multiply; differences between the attitudes of Member States towards social protection measures are more marked than ever, especially as the UK has become one of the world's low-tax economies.

Economic issues relating to the 'four freedoms' continue to have social consequences, and freedom of movement of people is particularly likely to exacerbate these problems. An example is the recent friction between the German government and the UK, which centred on the use being made of British sub-contractors and workers in the German construction industry. British workers, whether paid the same or less than German workers, were infuriating the host nation by not paying tax and national insurance contributions, whilst their German colleagues paid far in excess of British levels. The German government perceived this as a time bomb for the British, but could not secure agreement at European level for legislation to deal with the problem, and were reduced to using national legislation.

Enlargement has also given more prominence to the perceptions of Scandinavian countries, and their views about the relationship between the economy and social protection are not in agreement with UK government thinking.

UK citizens have already benefited considerably from policies developed at European level, although they may not be fully aware of how these have affected their lives. Environmental improvements like clean beaches and reduction in pollution by vehicle emissions, quality of drinking water, reductions in tobacco advertising, and equal employment rights for women and expectant mothers are a few of the results of membership of the European Union. Measures likely to be popular with the public tend not to be attributed by the media (or the government) to European policies and legislation. Others, such as metrication, are seen as unpopular by the press and TV and presented as unwelcome impositions. It is noticeable that many of the measures perceived as benefits are related to quality of life rather than concerned purely with economics.

Summary points

1 There is a strongly held view in the Union that economic union cannot be achieved without a corresponding social union, and that the Union's economic strength and prosperity in the world arena will depend on its capacity to build an open active and fair society which can mobilize energies and talents and improve the quality of life. The counter-view, held strongly by recent British Conservative governments, is that social legislation hampers competitiveness and economic buoyancy, and should rest largely in the national domain.

2 The Union's social aspirations to date are encapsulated in the Social Charter Action Programme and the Social Chapter of the Maastricht Treaty (1992). Because of the lack of consensus on social union, real progress has been slow and subject to opt-out, as far as the UK is concerned.

3 The two sides of industry are perceived by the Commission as being important players on the European policy front. They are seen as social partners, not as natural opponents.

4 Since Maastricht, the main lines of development have been set out in the White Paper, *European Social Policy – A Way Forward for the Union* (for the period 1995–99). This makes a crucial link between social measures and competitiveness, and between health promotion and economic and social prosperity.

5 Health has moved to occupy a place within the EU's social policy. Starting from the control of hazards, the Union's activities now extend to action against major diseases and health promotion. Harmonization of objectives across Member States includes a high level of health protection.

6 Most significantly, Article 129 of the Union Treaty gives a degree of legal competence to the European Commission in the area of public health. This is a modest beginning, hedged about with respect for the principle of subsidiarity, but it provides a foundation for strengthening the European Parliament's commitment to establishing a health policy for the Community.

7 A limited framework for action in the field of public health has been built on Article 129, with a central theme of

supporting and co-ordinating actions within Member States on a range of major issues which are common to the Community as a whole. In particular, it makes provision for large-scale analysis of the cost-effectiveness of measures, the formulation of new measures, and networks to facilitate communication between researchers and practitioners across the Union.

8 The Commission is conscious of the need to tread warily, because the funding and delivery of health care is primarily a matter for the Member States. But as one of the fundamental building blocks of a well-functioning and successful society, it cannot be left aside.

9 One of the four freedoms of the Union – freedom of movement – actually presents a risk and challenge in health terms. On the positive side, the free movement of health professionals is intended to be an important dimension in the development of a Union programme on public health.

References and further reading

The European Public Health Alliance. (1995). *Public health and the EU – an Overview*. EPHA. (See the Resource section for the EPHA address.)

Normand, C. and Vaughan, J. P. (eds) (1993). *Europe Without Frontiers. The Implications for Health*. John Wiley & Sons.

Social Chapter of the Maastricht Treaty. (1992). The Office for Official Publications of the European Communities.

Social Chapter Action Programme. COM. (89) 568 final. Commission of the European Communities.

Treaty of European Union. (1992). The Office for Official Publications of the European Communities.

5

Progress is bad for your health ... other European policies and their health implications

Aims of this Chapter

In this chapter, we aim to:
- outline the health implications of some other European policy areas and set health issues within a more global context;
- focus on certain areas like the environment and work;
- detail some of the legislation passed;
- explain the conflicts of interest and obstacles to progress;
- describe some of the research work and networking being undertaken.

The environment is not a marginal consideration on the periphery of economic reality – it intimately affects the health, quality of life and future of every European citizen. There is no shortage of scientific data on the ills being suffered by the environment. The challenge rests with us all; whether as policy makers or planners, banks or businesses, enterprises or private individuals. Public and private sectors must co-operate.

Yannis Paleokrassas, European Commissioner with responsibility for the environment in 1993 (Protecting our Environment, Europe on the Move series, 1993.)

Take a deep breath – if you dare

It has taken us until almost the end of the second millennium to realize that the health and well-being of all living things on the planet is linked inextricably to the environment, which in turn is in a delicate balance, sensitive to both natural and artificial disruption. We have learned this the hard way; man-made pollutants have caused illness to many thousands of people and resulted in enormous costs, both indirect and direct, to health services. In addition, damage caused to animal and plant life is likely to have repercussions for a long time in the future, especially in terms of the food chain.

We have also created working and living environments and lifestyles which have resulted in a rash of health problems of their own. Yet the growth of the world population, together with the decline in traditional industries and widespread economic recession, requires that our economies grow and develop to meet increasing needs. New technologies create possibilities for development but also present potential problems, some of which only emerge with widespread use. In turn, these advances create expectations, the most general being that progress will continue, and that the conveniences of modern life (at least in the West) are not only here to stay but will be superseded by even better things to come.

Concern for the environment has become a major political and consumerist force, yet at the same time, employment creation and economic regeneration is a priority for virtually all developed countries. In the past, these have been regarded as virtually incompatible. The success of the Green lobby in awakening the genuine concern of many ordinary citizens and voters has ensured that the political will exists to find a way of marrying up the two. At European level, environmental issues were seen as particularly important; the river polluted by one country's industry will not become instantly clean when it crosses a state boundary. The lesson of Chernobyl was a hard one, but it demonstrated that pollutants of all kinds are no respecters of national borders.

The European Community has long been concerned with environmental issues and has had environmental programmes since 1973. A range of directives on environmental protection have been issued and Article 130r of the Maastricht Treaty explicitly states that 'protecting human health' is an objective of European environmental policy. The Commission is currently implementing its Fifth Action Programme for the environment (1993–97) and is taking a different line in this to previous programmes. The policy change is reflected in the title *Towards Sustainability* (Com (92) 23 final), and addresses the whole issue of management of growth, a major concern at the 1992 Earth Summit. The aim is to embed an integrated approach to management of the environment, rather than tackling specific problems in a more piecemeal way as before. 'Sustainable development' is a central objective and the Action programme sets targets to be met by the year 2000 in the areas of industry, energy, agriculture, transport and tourism.

The Commission's view was that the environment is a fundamental concern, not only in relation to internal policies – that is, for the Member States – but in terms of external relations with other countries. The EU must therefore work internationally and seek to encourage sustainable, responsible development, if the environment globally is not to suffer. Yannis Paleokrassas, Environment Commissioner in 1993, voiced the perception that environmental issues were central to economic and social policies: 'Integrating the environment into the heartland of our economic policy is as important as any of the Community's policy commitments ... Any development which is unsustainable will prove to have been no development at all.' (Europe on the Move series,1993).

The problem, of course, is that environmental issues are popular with consumers only if they do not involve potential reductions in immediate levels of comfort and changes to lifestyles. Central heating may be using up fossil fuels and also be responsible for health problems, directly and indirectly (increases in house mites and respiratory illnesses as well as the polluting effects of fossil fuel power stations) but none of us wants to do without it. The same is true of other advances; employers may now be aware of the potential dangers of working with visual display units (VDUs) and computer keyboards, but they are here to stay.

The European Commission and the Parliament have both made clear their concern that new developments and pan-

European initiatives should take account of environmental issues at an early stage. Many EU-funded developmental projects require that the environmental and/or socio-economic factors of new developments be taken into account and their impact assessed prior to implementation. This at least shows an awareness of the issues and a sensitivity to them, but it remains to be seen whether these considerations are really allowed to stand in the way of economic growth. Past developments such as industrialization and mechanization have revealed themselves to be juggernauts which crushed opposition and left both human and environmental casualties in their wake.

Article 129 of the Maastricht Treaty requires the Commission to identify the health implications in EU policy areas across the board, and on the 29 May 1995, the Commission duly produced its first full report to the Council, the Parliament and the Economic and Social Committee (COM (95) 196 final).

European policy areas with health implications

Many policy areas are included in the Commission's report and some of the main ones are outlined below. This section is not a summary of the report, however; additional information has been included on other relevant EU legislation where this is relevant to health care. (The evolution of European social policy is described in the previous chapter.)

The **free movement of goods** is one of the primary aims of the Single Market and arguably (at least for 'free market' governments like the UK's) the most important benefit of the European Union. European legislation requires that health considerations are taken into account in this policy area and the legislation is particularly extensive in relation to dangerous substances. The public is probably unaware of the nature and extent of this legislation or believes that national legislation would anyway be sufficient protection from 'foreign' imports of dubious quality. The latter view may be true in certain cases, but it is impossible for every item imported from another source to be checked thoroughly on entry to the UK, and people purchase items whilst travelling which they then bring home and use. An example of 'unknown' legislation is the control of the use of nickel via a directive of 1994, which protects consumers against its potential dangers, for example, in jewellery manufacture.

Pharmaceutical products have been the focus of legislation since 1965. Controls are now strict and extensive and innovatory medicinal products will be subject to central authorization from the European Medicines Evaluation Agency, the EMEA. (Conventional medicines have a separate, decentralized procedure based on mutual recognition by the Member States.) The intention is that all EU citizens will have early access to medicinal products, and that there will be no national differences in safety evaluation or conditions of use. In addition to the 'free movement' legislation, there are controls on the advertising of medicines and on the minimum standards of information provided on their packaging and on information leaflets (Directive 92/27/EEC). Product legislation specifies that information provided about medicines must be clear and in terms which the patient can understand. Information must be included about the recommended dose and suitability, frequency of use and the potential side-effects, as well as a list of ingredients and the manufacturer's details.

Despite this breadth of legislation, there is no harmonization system in place for medicines and their use is felt to be too closely linked to national health systems to enable this to happen. Different medicines are used in different Member States, though some may simply have different names and be identical in other respects. Costs vary enormously, and some medicines which are available only on prescription in one Member State may be sold in a pharmacy in the neighbouring country, and may be available in supermarkets elsewhere.

The pharmaceutical industry has been accused of secrecy and of using commercial confidentiality in a way that excludes both health care professionals and patients from accessing information about drugs, which may be withdrawn from use without any explanation. The USA has legislation on freedom of information which does not permit this level of secrecy, and consumer groups are hoping that the commitment of the EU to openness will ensure that information about medicinal products will become more easily and widely available in the future. A small beginning will be made by the new Agency, the EMEA, which is to produce an assessment summary for medicines approved via the new centralized system. However, this will only be available to 'interested persons' and will cover the minority of products which are the responsibility of the EMEA; the decentralized system covers the rest, and information on the products approved will be provided at the discretion of the national agency concerned. This is hardly a revolution in openness and freedom of information.

European legislation on **medical devices** establishes a consistent approach to safety standards in design, manufacture and marketing of products. The directives cover 'active implantable medical devices' (Directive 90/385/EEC) which is now in force and 'medical devices' (93/42/EEC), which range from rubber catheters to anaesthesia machines. The latter will not be fully in force until June 1998. More recently, a new directive was proposed on '*in vitro* medical devices', and this is still at the proposal stage at the time of writing. The intention here is to harmonize the market and to ensure safeguards. This is obviously an extremely important area, and UK readers will remember that problems were experienced with blood bags in 1994 which had serious consequences. Blood bags are, in fact, covered by the 'medical devices' directive.

Energy is a major EU policy area – although there is still no structured European Energy Policy in place – which has implications for health, not only in terms of air quality and sulphur dioxide emissions but for the long-term effects of fossil fuels and chlorofluorocarbons (CFCs) in creating global warming and in the damage done to the ozone layer. A relatively short time ago, there was general scoffing at the idea of increases in cases of skin cancer due to ozone damage, and even more hilarity at the thought of malaria finding its way to northern Europe. Now energy policies are being taken more seriously; however, the hole in the ozone layer was found to be even bigger in 1995 than previously, and there is no sign that the developing countries will be more responsible in their use of energy than those of the 'old world' or the 'new world'.

However, legislation is only effective when it is properly implemented and the European directives on sulphur dioxide emissions from power plants are said to have been unevenly implemented and policed across the EU.

The Commission's aim is towards rational and efficient energy use which improves the quality of life. **Transport** policy, with its clear links with energy policy, has considerable public health implications. Air quality has given cause for concern in recent years, not only in urban population centres but in rural parts of the EU. Combined with other atmospheric pollutants, vehicle emissions have caused widespread poor air quality and this almost certainly accounts for increases in respiratory diseases such as asthma. The EU's transport strategy aims to develop public transport and improve technology in order to reduce pollution, as well as to encourage measures designed to reduce the need for travel (such as use of 'virtual' sites, homeworking etc.). The first directive on motor vehicle emissions dates back to 1970 and has been updated several times since, with the latest update in 1993. Further proposals can be expected in the future. At the same time, the freedom of movement and dismantling of barriers brought about by the Single Market are more likely to increase traffic then reduce it.

The Common Transport Policy actually addresses health protection requirements mainly via measures to ensure safety and reduce accidents. Road accident rates vary considerably between Member States but the Commission is also concerned with safety of other forms of transport.

Agriculture continues to be a problem for the EU, which still struggles to find a form of support for the industry which is acceptable to farmers, governments and consumers. The over-use of fertilizers and pesticides has caused concerns, especially when these have drained into rivers and reservoirs, and there are issues here for food safety too. The Commission's aim is to strike a balance between agriculture and the rural environment, encouraging rural development of various kinds and responsible use of natural resources. In addition, there is considerable legislation relating to animal health and hygiene and plant health which aims to ensure that this stage of the food chain is free from health hazards. **Food**

and food production and sales are also subjects for European legislation, ranging from directives on permitted additives to frozen food and food hygiene generally.

One topic familiar to the British over recent years is the controversial one of **water quality**. As far back as 1975, the European Commission has been concerned with the quality of drinking water and produced directives on water intended for human consumption. Evidence linking lead intake with brain damage in children has now caused the Commission to propose new limits on lead in drinking water (i.e. from 50 to 10 microgrammes per litre). This is a particular concern in some parts of the UK where there are still extensive lead mains water pipes, as well as household pipework. Pollution of groundwater by agriculture, industry or sites used for dumping waste has also caused concern, and the problem of nitrates in water was tackled by a EC directive of 1991 (91/676). Bathing water has perhaps received the most publicity in recent years when several of the UK's most popular beaches were found to be in breach of recommended levels of pollution. This controversy was compounded by the fact that Member State governments had been asked to produce lists of beaches, and the UK's definition of a beach was so narrow that we apparently had very few, despite being an island. Other countries, for example Luxembourg, which has no coastline, had included lakeside and riverside beaches in their lists.

The world of work

It is almost a cliché now that a healthy economy is one which is not only financially prosperous in terms of its balance of payments and national debt, but which integrates its population in economic activity. The economic integration of groups like the disabled, women and disadvantaged people has long been part of European policy and 'social exclusion' is recognized not merely as a social problem but one which impacts on the state as a whole.

Patterns of work and the nature of work itself have changed considerably in recent years. Change has become normal. This does not mean that the experience of change is welcomed or even accepted, and the challenges it brings are frequently perceived as threats, problems and anxieties. Working conditions in the past – even the recent past – were fraught with dangers such as contact with toxic substances like asbestos and insufficient safeguards against industrial accident and injury. New technologies and ways of working may hold their own threats which workers have yet to fully experience.

The European Foundation for the Improvement of Living and Working Conditions

Health and safety in the workplace is often seen as a rather narrow area of activity and one which is of little interest to many health care professionals. The European Commission takes a rather broader view and sets work within the context of people's lives to assess its real impact. The organization responsible for much developmental and co-ordination work on this is the European Foundation for the Improvement of Living and Working Conditions. The Foundation was established in 1975 and is an autonomous body of the EU. It has a four-year rolling programme which currently runs from 1993–96. Its broad aims and the areas where it feels it can make a contribution are:

- improving the health and well-being of European workers and citizens;
- increasing economic and social cohesion and fighting against the exclusion of disadvantaged groups;
- maintaining the move towards a sustainable and integrated development of social, economic and ecological aspects of living and working conditions.

The Foundation has evolved a series of key principles for its work which include an integrated approach to living and working conditions and the environment. Other principles highlight participation of those involved, priority being given to preventative actions, and equality of opportunity and treatment.

The work of the Foundation includes managing projects on health and safety and as a result of one of these, it maintains the HASTE database (Health and Safety in Europe). This developed from a project undertaken in 1989–90 on identifying risk factors for workers. The database aims to catalogue information systems across the EU and beyond (the Czech Republic and Norway are included) to identify health and safety risks and determine indicators for possible preventative measures.

Other published reports on project work include such topics as:

- Family care of the elderly;
- Preventing racism at the workplace;
- Identification and assessment of occupational health strategies in Europe;
- Ill-health and workplace absenteeism – initiatives for prevention;
- Innovative workplace action for health;
- The electronic home: telemedicine and telehealth.

The Foundation also publishes a review of issues relating to health and safety at work, *Euro Review*, which reports on the findings of European research projects. This evolved from work carried out in preparation for the new European Agency for Health and Safety at Work, and the concern that, though considerable research was underway on health and safety issues, dissemination of results was often insufficiently widespread. The Foundation therefore organized a Euro Research Network of contacts within EU countries, the Commission and others, such as the USA and the International Labour Office in Geneva, to exchange information about ongoing research. It also undertook project work on health risks in certain sectors and selected the meat processing industry and hospitals as pilot areas. The risks examined were the traditional, physical ones such as industrial injuries and exposure to chemicals, plus 'newer' problems such as time pressures, workload and stress.

Health risks in the hospital working environment

The research project studied hospitals in 10 European Union countries. Researchers found the sector to have considerable economic weight and the work force represented 2.9–5.5 per cent of the national working populations in the countries concerned. The majority of workers are female, have had an intermediate or low education and are employed full-time. Though a high degree of medical technology was found, most of the work still involves physical hard labour. A great variety of materials are used and a wide range of equipment. Five main trends were identified, specifically:

- an increase in expenses coupled with economic constraints and the need to reduce costs;
- ongoing development of high technology equipment;
- an increase in intensive care;
- introduction of new management concepts such as total quality management;
- implementation of EC occupational health and safety directives.

In all the countries studied, the sector had undertaken various improvements to working conditions but still experienced occupational health and safety problems. There was consensus on four risk factors: musculoskeletal loads, biological agents, chemical substances and deviant working hours. Another three risk factors were identified in the majority of countries: relations with clients and the public (i.e. violence at work, and dealing with pain and dying people), division of work and job content (i.e. monotonous work, lack of control, and autonomy) and relations with colleagues (isolation, lack of teamwork, and support). These risk factors were thought to contribute to stress and 'burn-out'. Some groups were more at risk than others, and researchers identified three main risk groups. These were nurses, who make up 11–44 per cent of hospital workers, service and tradeworkers (2–30 per cent) and nurse assistants and apprentices (10–27 per cent). Laboratory workers and anaesthetists were also seen as risk groups.

The study recommended that hospitals should give priority to making improvement in four main areas:

- The physical work environment, particularly in relation to musculoskeletal loads, hospital agents and chemical substances;
- The organizational work environment, so as to provide work schedules which provide a healthy balance between workload and recovery, and organization of work to improve working relations between various occupational categories;
- The social work environment, both in terms of relations with clients and with colleagues. Issues include violence at work, new nursing concepts, and staff training;
- The health and safety policy, which should operate for all staff and focus on prevention.

Policy options were also suggested for sectoral organizations and for national governments. These results and recommendations are taken from *Working Conditions at Sectoral Level in Europe: Hospital Activities* (1995). Another useful source of information is the European Centre for Work and Society, which is an independent non-profit making organization. It aims to 'aid the overall development of work-related policies and to assess their social and economic impact in a European context'.

Conclusions

Wherever human beings, and living things for that matter, exist and engage in activity, there will be implications for their health and well-being. The complex interactions between environments and activities are becoming better understood, but knowledge and understanding does not always lead to improving action. National policies have demonstrated that economic prosperity today has often taken precedence over environmental safeguards or even health considerations, and the acid rain falling in one environmentally aware country may be the product of its neighbour's industry. The principle of the polluter being made to pay is certainly an advance on the past, but in practice it may prove difficult to apply. Nevertheless improvements which result in better standards of health are to be welcomed, however cautious they may be. The consideration being given to the impact of new technologies on workers is one such advance; it may do no more in the short term than ensure slight ameliorations in working conditions but at least it ensures that people become more aware of risks, that employers are more aware of their responsibilities and employees of their rights and the individual safeguards available to them.

In addition, the European framework within which these policies operate is likely to have a beneficial effect, especially with the enlargement of the Union to include Sweden and Finland, as the Scandinavian countries have a reputation for social and environmental awareness and responsibility. Within the Union, the opportunities for networking and exchanging good practice are enormous, and there are also possibilities for innovatory improvements made in one sector to be more easily transferred to another. An appreciation of the global picture of European policy, and the way that one policy area interacts with another, is essential if this is to take place.

Summary points

1 Public health, including its cost and the demands placed upon its services, is linked inextricably to environmental conditions, which ought therefore to be a concern for the health care professional.
2 The European Union's environmental programme, *Towards Sustainability*, seeks to integrate consideration of environmental implications into the early stages of policy development on all fronts. As a result, proposals are routinely vetted for the protection of public health.
3 The free movement of goods, including dangerous substances, pharmaceutical products and medical devices, energy supply and use, transportation, agricultural production and food processing, and water supply are all subject to EU regulations in the interests of public health. These are often cautious and limited in the face of other considera-

tions, but are still to be welcomed as a form of progress. They are helping to ensure a growing awareness of environmental risks, rights and responsibilities.

4 A broader, more environmentally conscious view of health and safety in the workplace is emerging, centred on the European Foundation for the Improvement of Living and Working Conditions and its work in managing projects, reviewing research and encouraging information exchange through networks.

5 There are some grounds for optimism. The Scandinavian countries bring to the Union a strong reputation for social and environmental awareness and responsibility; within the Union the opportunities for exchanging good practice are enormous, and there are possibilities for transferring innovatory improvements.

References and further reading

Protecting our Environment, Europe on the Move series. (1993). Commission of the European Communities.

Report from the Commission to the Council, the European Parliament and the Economic and Social Committee on the integration of health protection requirements in Community policies. COM (95) 196 final. Commission of the European Communities.

Towards Sustainability, A European Community Programme of Policy and Action in relation to the Environment and Sustainable Development. COM (92) 23 final. Vol 2, Commission of the European Communities.

Verschuren, R., de Groot, S. N. and Nossent, S. (1995). Project of the *Working Conditions at Sectoral Level in Europe: Hospital Activities.* European Foundation for the Improvement of Living and Working Conditions.

6

Public health – the challenges for Europe

Aims of this Chapter

In this chapter, we aim to:
- highlight the major health issues facing European Union countries;
- outline the major causes of mortality and morbidity in Europe;
- explain the nature of the relationship between the European Union and the World Health Organization (WHO);
- consider the various approaches towards improving the health of the nation;
- suggest where the future direction of health policies might lie for EU countries.

For decades, health seemed a relatively isolated and undisturbed field. Today it is perhaps the sector most affected by the current political and economic crises. Health has become a favourite theme of the mass media and public opinion, and is therefore at the centre of political debates that influence the choice of policies.

Health in Europe. 1994

Health trends in Europe – a brief overview

Health systems in Europe differ greatly, not only in terms of organization and structure but in terms of the culture and traditions which have developed around them. For example, attitudes to what the British might call 'alternative' medicine differ significantly from one Member State to another, as does drug consumption in relation to certain diseases. There are also significant differences in lifestyle and working environment which have health implications and result in variations in cancers of various kinds, heart disease and other conditions. At the same time, trends are emerging across the EU in relation to health care issues which are shared in all European countries, although no attempt is likely to be made in the foreseeable future to harmonize health care or to try to put in place a European health service.

People generally are enjoying better health than in the past, with higher standards of hygiene, nutrition and living and working conditions. This is reflected in rates for life expectancy, infant mortality and average population height. Ironically, the decline in communicable diseases has been balanced to a large extent by the increase in lifestyle-related diseases such as those linked to smoking and drinking. Traditionally, women suffered lower rates of smoking-related and stress-related diseases than men, but now the rates are converging.

Health costs are rising in all Member States despite efforts to control spending. The major factors are:

- increased life expectancy which results in larger numbers of older people, who are disproportionate users of health care services;
- new technologies for diagnosis and treatment;
- diseases and conditions relating to the working environment, such as stress;
- rising expectations of health and standards of fitness.

It is ironic that all but one of the above (i.e. work-related conditions) actually represent the problems of success for health and welfare services.

Most European governments are faced with a dilemma on health spending and welfare generally. Although expenditure will continue to rise and is unlikely to be balanced by economic growth, there appears to be little support for higher taxation and social insurance costs in most countries. The inevitable reduction in public spending is therefore likely to result in an increase in the private insurance and health care sector.

The state of Europe's health – a level playing field?

One of the objectives of the European Union is to help to raise standards, both economic and social, in those countries or regions which are less developed than the European average. The intention is to create the 'level playing field' so beloved of media commentators and politicians, which will enable ease of movement and the creation of stable and thriving economies and communities within the overall, global framework of the Union. This will be achieved in a variety of ways: by funded programmes which provide assistance for capital projects, or training or pump-prime innovatory work, by legislation to create a common legal framework across the EU, and by initiatives of various kinds which aim to spread best practice, encourage collaboration and raise standards across the Union.

One of these is the publication of an annual *Report on the state of health in the European Community*. The first of these was produced by the European Commission in July 1995 (COM (95) 357 final). Based on data available in 1994, the report describes the major health trends and issues in the then 12 Member States, and the snapshot it provides, though limited, will help to enable comparisons to be made in the future. Information for the report was taken from a wide variety of sources, including EUROSTAT (the EU's statistical office), the OECD (Organization for Economic Co-operation and Development), WHO's Health for All database and national government Health for All reports, together with other reports and scientific data. Disease-specific interest groups also provided material, such as the International Agency for Research on Cancer (IARC), the European Centre for Epidemiological Monitoring of AIDS and the

European Registration of Congenital Anomalies and Twins (EUROCAT).

More recently, the Commission issued a *Communication and draft decision on a Community action programme on health monitoring*. This is a five-year programme, running from 1997–2001, and focuses on four main areas: identification and establishment of health indicators and data at both EU and Member State levels, a national/international data collection and dissemination network, analysis of health indicators and trends and dissemination of information (COM (95) 449 final, 16 October 1995).

The inclusion of the Public Health Article in the Union Treaty legitimizes action at EU level, albeit of a limited nature, and many health care practitioners feel this to be long overdue. Standards in health care in the EU taken as an average are apparently acceptable – for example, Europe has a very low infant mortality rate and a high life expectancy – but closer inspection at Member State and regional level reveals considerable variation. The need for a level playing field must be as urgent in health care as in industry and commerce, and a great deal could be achieved by working collaboratively at EU level.

Cardiovascular diseases are a major cause of death in Europe, accounting for about half of all deaths and a high percentage of permanent disability. These diseases are also responsible for a huge proportion of health care costs and represent an enormous burden on the budgets of all Member States. Lifestyle factors are well-known to play a key role in the onset and development of cardiovascular diseases, including smoking, poor nutrition and low levels of activity leading to high blood pressure, high levels of cholesterol and obesity. Other causes of death also relate to lifestyle, as Table 1, showing leading causes of death by age and sex, illustrates.

Experience gained via World Health Organization programmes dating back to the 1970s indicated that planned and properly co-ordinated intersectoral efforts could lower the risk factors. This needs to be done at the level of agencies working together at strategic levels, and within an increasingly global society, must be done at a global level. A good example of this

Table 1. Leading causes of death by age and sex in the European Community

Age (years)	Male	Female
Under 1	Hypoxia, birth asphyxia and other respiratory conditions	Hypoxia, birth asphyxia and other respiratory conditions
1–4	Motor vehicle accidents	Congenital anomalies of heart and circulatory system
5–9	Motor vehicle accidents	Motor vehicle accidents
10–14	Motor vehicle accidents	Motor vehicle accidents
15–19	Motor vehicle accidents	Motor vehicle accidents
20–24	Motor vehicle accidents	Motor vehicle accidents
28–29	Motor vehicle accidents	Motor vehicle accidents
30–34	Motor vehicle accidents	Suicide
35–39	Suicide	Breast cancer
40–44	Acute myocardial infarction	Breast cancer
45–49	Acute myocardial infarction	Breast cancer
50–54	Acute myocardial infarction	Breast cancer
55–59	Acute myocardial infarction	Breast cancer
60–64	Acute myocardial infarction	Breast cancer
65–69	Acute myocardial infarction	Acute myocardial infarction
70–74	Acute myocardial infarction	Acute myocardial infarction
75–79	Acute myocardial infarction	Acute myocardial infarction
80–84	Acute myocardial infarction	Acute cerebrovascular disease
Over 85	Disease of pulmonary circulation and other cardiopathies	Disease of pulmonary circulation and other cardiopathies

Source: World Health Organization
Taken from the Commission *Communication on the framework for action in the field of public health*, COM (93) 559 final. Reproduced with the kind permission of the Commission of the European Communities.

is food quality and hygiene, including nutrition. This is also a major factor in relation to cancer, which is the second largest cause of mortality in the EU. Again, there are wide variations in incidence and types of cancer found throughout Europe, and only a small proportion of these variations are likely to be genetically related. For example, the incidence of death from breast cancer is high in the UK, Denmark and Ireland, and low in Greece, Portugal and Spain. Portugal and Italy have higher instances of cancers of the stomach, and deaths related to male smoking (via various cancers) are particularly high in the Netherlands and Belgium. (Source: *Rapid Reports: Population and Social Conditions*, 1993). Smoking-related cancer rates are often at variance with the actual number of smokers in the population because there is a time factor of 15–20 years before the disease develops or becomes apparent, so that it may not be perceived to be a health problem by governments until too late. This is another area where experience could be usefully shared between agencies and governments at a pan-European or international level, and the European Commission has done much to facilitate this, via the *Europe Against Cancer* campaign.

However, although it is now universally recognized that lifestyle factors are thought to be vitally important in health protection, government intervention has been extremely low-key throughout Europe. Part of the problem is that though the message from health care professionals and researchers is clear, tensions and conflicts exist within the political and industrial worlds which result in a lack of determined action. Health lobbies are traditionally poorly funded and supported, whilst agrochemical, agricultural lobbies and food processing lobbies pack much more of a punch, and also threaten governments with hefty job losses – a deciding factor in terms of political health, if not the health of the nation (a good example of this is the tobacco industry, as described later in this chapter).

Differences also exist with regard to cancer survival rates. The Eurocare study, which is following 800 000 cancer patients in 11 European (not EU) countries, is compiling data on the treatment and survival rates of patients five years after diagnosis. Cancer patients in Finland, Switzerland and the Netherlands had the best survival rates with the worst being recorded in Poland and Estonia. England and Scotland scored badly for men and women with stomach and colon cancers, and for cancers of the cervix, breast, lung and ovaries in women.

Communicable diseases remain a major health concern throughout the European Union. The most high-profile example of these is perhaps the AIDS epidemic, but in fact problems are being experienced in a number of countries by an apparent resurgence of the 'old' diseases which many people believed to be virtually extinct in the developed world. The most persistent of these is tuberculosis, which may be assisted by waves of migration due to war and economic factors. In addition, increases in homelessness and overcrowding are likely to facilitate the spread of the disease.

Mental health problems appear to be another area of concern across the EU, with rates of youth suicide on the increase in some Member States and rises in consumption of tranquillizers and anti-depressants. Homicide and purposeful injury also appears to be generally increasing.

International co-operation

Until the Public Health Article introduced into the Union Treaty gave some legal competence in the area of health to the European institutions, the main international body with responsibility for public health matters was the World Health Organization. Created in 1948, the WHO has a membership of 180 countries and enables the health professions of members to exchange knowledge and experience with the aim of attaining for all citizens of the world a level of health that will permit them to lead a socially and economically productive life.

The WHO Regional Office for Europe is one of six such offices and is situated in Copenhagen. The WHO's framework for action is encapsulated in the Health for All by the Year 2000 policy, which focuses clearly on primary care via Target 26. This states: 'by the year 2000 all member states (i.e. of WHO) should have developed and be implementing policies that ensure universal access to health services of quality, based on primary care and supported by secondary and tertiary care.' (World Health Organization, 1992).

Although the institutions of the EU and the WHO have previously had no structured history of close collaboration, the situation is likely to change in the future. The Commission's *Communication on the framework for action in the field of public health* makes explicit the need to work with other international organizations, and in particular the WHO, and clearly identifies the benefits of mutual collaboration. European institutions in particular could benefit from the extensive networks established by the WHO as well as the data it holds. And though the Health for All initiative has had some impact, the work of the WHO must inevitably suffer from the unevenness of commitment and resourcing which affects all voluntary initiatives; a framework for action embracing a bloc of 15 countries could provide an unprecedented opportunity for collaboration on health problems and solutions.

The problems facing Europe's health policy makers – can pan-European action really help?

The common problems being faced by most, if not all, EU countries call for transferable solutions to be devised. The point has already been made that there is a need for the various agencies to work together, interdependently, for the maximum impact to be achieved, and the European Union provides the obvious framework for this. The Commission have taken a lead where possible, with certain key areas having been identified as those which would benefit from action at European Union level. The recently issued *Report on the integration of health protection requirements in Community policies* (COM (95) 196 final) also attempted to provide a survey of the various Community policies with a health care aspect or implication. The report illustrates how health-related issues have been tackled within various programmes and policy areas, such as transport and agriculture, as well as in more obvious ones like safety of goods.

The Commission's strategy for implementing the Maastricht Treaty provisions relating to health were set out in its *Communication on the framework for action in the field of public health* (COM (93) 559 final), as already discussed. This identified the problems regarded as 'major scourges' and gave careful consideration to the practical possibilities for intervention and also to the potential value of pan-European activity (Table 2). The priorities identified are being targeted for action, or have already been the subject of developmental or demonstration work.

The interdependence of these factors needs to be stressed,

Table 2.   Identification of 'major scourges' in the European Community

Disease/health problem	Standardized death rates per 100 000 or incidences per 100 000 (estimates)	Costs for health services (and other costs e.g. absenteeism)	Practical possibilities for prevention	Community added value (opportunities for intervention)	'Major scourges' (major health problems)	Previous Community public health action
Cancer	337	***	***	****	****	****
Cancer of colon	29					
Lung cancer	42					
Digestive organs	62					
Breast cancer	33					
Prostate cancer	19					
Diseases of the circulatory system	338	****	***	****	****	**
Hypertensive disease	16					
Acute myocardial infarction	90					
Cerebrovascular disease	90					
Ischaemic heart disease	137					
Respiratory diseases		***	***	***	***	**
Bronchitis, emphysema, asthma	17	***	****	***	*	**
Congenital abnormalities	5	***	****	***	*	**
Perinatal conditions	5	****	****	****	****	**
Accidents (including poisoning)	51	***	****	****	****	***
Motor vehicle accidents	15	****	***	***	***	***
Drug and alcohol abuse		***	****	****	****	***
Musculoskeletal problems		****	***	***	***	**
Visual problems		**	**	*	*	*
Auditory problems		*	**	*	*	*
Mental disorders		****	**	*	***	*
Suicides	13	***	***	***	***	***
Nutrition-related disorders, including diabetes, dental caries		***	***	***	**	***

Table 2. (*continued*)

Disease/health problem	Standardized death rates per 100 000 or incidences per 100 000 (estimates)	Costs for health services (and other costs e.g. absenteeism)	Practical possibilities for prevention	Community added value (opportunities for intervention)	'Major scourges' (major health problems)	Previous Community public health action
AIDS	2.41 (incidence)					
Other communicables diseases,		***	****	****	***	***
e.g. Sexually transmitted diseases and tuberculosis		***	****	****	***	***
Childhood infections						
Measles	51 (incidence)	**	****	****	*	*
Rubella	26 (incidence)					
Other childhood infections						
Rare diseases, e.g. Thalassaemia, sickle-cell anaemia, rickets		*	***	***	**	*
Food-borne diseases e.g. salmonella poisoning		**	****	****	***	*

**** = High   *** = Medium   ** = Low   * = None.
Taken from the Commission *Communication on the framework for action in the field of public health*, COM (93) 559 final. Reproduced with the kind permission of the Commission of the European Communities.

and the reader should bear in mind the point already made that health care measures are vulnerable to pressure from other factors, such as the wider market economy. Some issues are explored below.

The ageing population: demographic nightmare or undervalued resource?

During the last three decades, the number of older people (aged 60 and upwards) has risen in the European Union from 46.5 to 68.6 million, an increase of almost 50 per cent excluding the three new Member States. (EUROSTAT, 1993/1).

The proportion of older people in the population will almost certainly continue to rise and current estimates indicate that there will be approximately twice as many older people in the EU by the year 2000 as there were in 1960. However, to think of older people as a uniform group would be quite inaccurate. Roughly half of them are aged between 60–69, about a third aged between 70–79 and only 17.4 per cent (11.9 million people) are over 80.

The steady rise in life expectancy is largely attributable to improvements in living and working conditions and advances in medical science. Women continue to benefit from increased life expectancy, with a woman aged 60 in 1988 having an average life expectancy of 82.5 years compared with her male counterpart's 78 years.

Figure 4 gives some indication of the differential between males and females, both at birth and at the age of 65. However, this is a European *average* and life expectancy does vary from one Member State to another (and indeed between regions). For example, in 1990, a Greek man of 60 had the highest male life expectancy in the EU, and his Irish counterpart the lowest.

Life expectancy, although it may be an indication of the general standard of living within a region or country, is a crude measure and tells us little about the *quality* of life. For older people, as for young families, improvements in living standards and amenities have coincided with changes in lifestyle which render them increasingly vulnerable to stress.

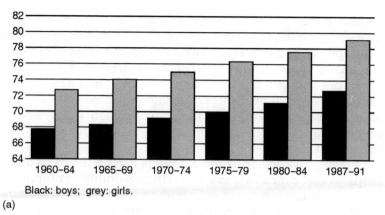

Black: boys; grey: girls.

(a)

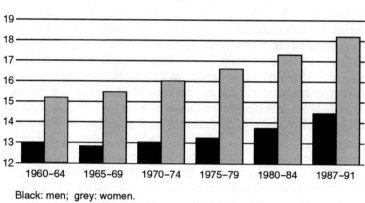

Black: men; grey: women.

(b)

Figure 4   Life expectancies of (a) girls and boys at birth, and (b) men and women at age 65. *Source*: EUROSTAT Yearbook 1995. Reproduced with kind permission of the Commission of the European Communities.

More older people are now living alone, not only as a result of one partner surviving the death of a spouse but because the extended family is no longer a feature of modern living, except in some ethnic minority groups. Another factor is the image most commonly presented of the elderly. We are all familiar with the idea of the weak and helpless old lady living in fear of muggers or the old man who does not know how to look after himself. Ours is not a society which values the elderly and old age is often viewed negatively, being associated with chronic illness, fear of crime, senility and a general state of dependence. The accuracy of this image is questionable; certainly health problems are likely to increase with the onset of old age, but many young disabled people overcome far greater infirmities and live full lives despite them. The fear of crime has been shown to be disproportionate to the amount of crime actually perpetrated against the individual; in other words, people's fear of crime is affecting their quality of life more than crime itself.

This negative image of the elderly is itself a threat to older people because it can act as a powerful self-fulfilling prophecy. Being frightened to go out increases isolation and reduces opportunities for interacting with other people in the community. Anxiety about lack of money, together with loneliness, can lead to depression and personal neglect. Lack of exercise or an inactive lifestyle can result in poor physical condition – and so on. The European Commission is well aware of the problems inherent in this situation and is trying to combat them by striking at the root of the negative image of old age. 1993 was designated as the 'Year of Older People and Solidarity between Generations' and used as a focus for a series of projects and activities which either presented a positive view of old age or explored ways of tackling some of the difficulties experienced by older people. Following the Year, a programme was set up to support other projects, and the theme is also present in some other EU funded programmes. The idea is to avoid presenting the elderly as a group which is separate to the rest of the population but as an integrated part of society, with a role to play as consumers, workers (should they wish to continue to be economically active), family members and participants in community life. Their experience and expertise is stressed, and one idea common to many projects is that of older people providing a valuable resource to local communities as repositories of local knowledge and skill. This is particularly in tune with the current interest in reviving community life and community spirit.

It is interesting to speculate on the possible effect a successful campaign of this nature might have on health budgets, could the public image, and the self-image, of the elderly genuinely change. Unfortunately, attitudes do not change overnight and the situation at present is that the growing numbers of older people require an increasing allocation of resources across all Member States. The problem is not only about money; many national governments need to reassess the human resources required to provide appropriate care and support services for older people, given their rate of increase in the population. By the year 2010, it is estimated that 14 per cent of the population will be under 25 as opposed to 18 per cent in 1990, yet the number of older people will have dramatically increased.

Free movement of people is also a factor, with most of those retired people who do move elsewhere tending to go south to take advantage of warmer climates. Already there are substantial colonies of retired Northern Europeans in certain favoured sites, mainly on the Mediterranean coast, and if this becomes a more widespread practice it will have implications in terms of social protection and medical services in those localities. Strategic planning and problem-solving at EU level is probably the only feasible way of tackling this issue.

Healthy lifestyles

Health promotion throughout the EU tends to be rather narrowly focused on issues such as smoking, substance misuse and human immunodeficiency virus (HIV) infection. Health promotion infrastructures which would benefit from modernization and reorganization are currently hampered by financial constraints, even though heath education has the potential to cut delivery costs substantially.

The creation of the WHO Healthy Cities initiative and the Healthy Schools projects have begun to change attitudes towards policies, structures and programmes which address broad lifestyle issues and create a kind of 'positive action' for health. Health issues in the past have actually been more concerned with illness and the prevention of disease; the focus more recently is on factors which promote well-being, rather than simply tackling ill-health. The European Union also agreed a Health Education programme worth 30 million ECU in June 1995, again with the aim of encouraging healthy living habits.

The creation of a healthy environment and lifestyle is clearly crucial to this policy and a whole range of contributory factors thereby come into play. The enormous range of EU directives and policy documents, especially in relation to issues like the environment, food production and working conditions, provide scope for the realization of such structural improvements. To the outsider, it is easy for the plethora of documentation to appear bureaucratic and over-regulatory, but the intention is for each piece of legislation and each policy document to have its place in the creation of a total global structure which benefits not just the European economy but ultimately the European citizen. The EU seeks to create a more prosperous economy without the worker exploitation which is, in the developing world, and has been, in the older industrial nations, a common feature of 'successful' economies. Health issues in their broadest sense are those which impact upon the mental, emotional and physical well-being of people.

An example of the European Commission's sensitivity to this is the push which is being given to the creation of an 'information society', based upon accessibility to information and know-how by means of information technology in its various forms. The Commission is keen to encourage the establishment and widespread acceptance of this, but at the same time is conscious of the possible effects and implications. Measures have been put in place to assess the socio-economic impact of the information society and its attendant initiatives (such as remote communication) and projects funded in relation to telematics development and exploitation must all address this issue. The Commission is clearly concerned that a rapid and radical change in working habits and increasing dependence on new technology could be accompanied by a range of information technology specific conditions, such as industrial injuries similar to those linked with the use of VDUs, or social and emotional effects which could have health implications.

The Commission's interventions are driven primarily by economic considerations and its health-related activities are largely viewed within this context (as indeed, are those of national governments). This renders some of its actions and policies open to question on health grounds, and aspects of the Common Agricultural Policy (CAP) are a good example of this.

The CAP and tobacco policies

The issue of state aid for industry and agriculture can be a particularly controversial area, both for national governments and for the European Union, and there is possibly no more controversial topic than aid for the tobacco industry. The EU provides substantial financial assistance for tobacco growers, who are generally based in the underdeveloped southern parts of Europe. Tobacco growers form part of the powerful agriculture lobby and are assisted by the cigarette manufacturing industry, which similarly is a powerful lobbying force. Member State governments also have a dual vested interest themselves, particularly those with tobacco producing areas and a high percentage of smokers in the population. Their desire to maintain the economic well-being of the regions concerned is compounded by an unwillingness to lose the revenues brought in by tobacco sales (not to mention the votes of the smokers in their electorate).

Conflicting with this is the enormous cost of tobacco-related diseases throughout the whole of the EU and the increasing amount of resource which is dedicated to treatment and patient care, smoking-related research and support for dependants of smokers, either during the course of chronic or terminal illness or following premature death. Of the 'top ten' cancers in the EC, lung cancer remains the commonest for men and was the leading male cancer in all former 12 Member States except for Portugal, where that position was occupied by stomach cancer. (Breast cancer is the most common for women.)

Nowhere is the irony (perhaps even cynicism) of this conflict better illustrated than in the policies and programmes of the EU, which on the one hand supports and finances the tobacco industry via the CAP, and on the other denounces the effects of tobacco consumption via the *Europe Against Cancer* campaign. The aim of the campaign is to substantially reduce cancer cases and one clearly identified means of achieving this is to discourage smoking. The Commission is acutely aware of this anomaly and has set up the Community Fund for tobacco research and information, with the aim of financing measures 'to discourage and provide information on smoking' and steer tobacco production towards the less harmful varieties. Attempts are also being made to persuade growers to change from tobacco to other crops. The fact remains that in 1994 the EU provided 1165 million ECU in tobacco subsidies and allocated a mere 15 million ECU to the Europe Against Cancer programme.

Most EU national governments have undertaken consumer campaigns to discourage smoking since the related health risks became apparent, but they have lacked coherence and critics say that they have also lacked real commitment. Smoking amongst young Europeans remains high and targets on reductions are unlikely to be met (the WHO target was that a minimum of 80 per cent of the population should be non-smoking by 1995, but the EC average 1987–89 was 64 per cent). Clearly, this is one area where European Union action could take a lead, but is hampered by the traditional supremacy of economic factors and the relative weakness and limited scope of the embryonic 'Social' Europe (the UK in particular, has in recent years stressed the role of the EU as a Single *Market*). Many health care professionals who are also committed pro-Europeans would like to see a strengthening of the role and competence of the European Commission in the field of health and social care, and an acceptance of the need for the current agriculture-driven policy, on tobacco production to give way to a health-driven policy, which would be unequivocally implemented. At present, economic considerations are clearly seen to continue to dominate the EU agenda.

Alcohol is also an issue here, though to a lesser extent, as the EU also supports this indirectly via subsidies, particularly to the wine industry. Again, the Commission notes that consumption of wine is falling and that the situation of growers is 'rather precarious', hence the need to avoid 'extreme measures' (COM (95) 196 final). Again, the conflict between economic considerations and health can be clearly recognized.

Drug misuse and associated problems

The use of psychoactive drugs has increased throughout the EU and evidence suggests that young people are experimenting with drugs more than ever before. The number of deaths recorded as drug-related in countries where monitoring takes place has also risen, which points to an increase in the use of so-called 'hard' drugs.

The EU is attempting to combat this in various ways, not least by initiatives which promote healthy lifestyles and educate young people in the dangers of drug misuse. In addition, efforts are being made to reduce the availability of illegal drugs by setting up collaborative policing and customs intelligence systems, in order to prevent drugs entering the EU from the country of origin or processing.

However, the lack of a pan-European policy on drugs is hampering progress, with a wide variation in attitudes towards drug use in the EU. Some Member States (the Netherlands, for example) have a liberal attitude towards drug misuse and a perception of addiction as illness, and have put strategies in place for dealing with the matter in a social and health-related context. In contrast, others (such as France) perceive the issue as almost entirely crime-related and have no social programmes in place, with the police as the only agency responsible for dealing with it; consequently the drug problem, and the user, become entirely criminalized. The issue has even threatened to disrupt progress made under the Schengen Agreement (whereby a group of Member States dismantled border controls and implemented total freedom of movement within their shared area), because of fears about free movement of drugs, especially from the Netherlands to France.

This is another area where clear advantages can be identified for a pan-European policy and strategy, but where national interests and attitudes are likely to dominate and hamper progress.

Sexual health

The incidence of HIV infection continues to increase throughout the EU, despite education programmes on safe sex being implemented by national governments. By 30 June 1994, a cumulative total of 108 872 AIDS cases had been reported in the then 12 Member States, including paediatric cases (Table 3). Three countries, France, Italy and Spain, accounted for over 72 per cent of reported cases.

Amongst those likely to have been infected by sexual transmission, statistics indicate an increase in the incidence of AIDS amongst heterosexuals (from 10.89 per cent in 1990 to 15.3 per cent in 1994) and a decrease in rates amongst homosexuals and bisexuals (from 39.3 to 32.2 per cent). The number of infected females remains relatively low amongst adolescent and adult age groups (15.29 per cent in 1994) but amongst paediatric cases, as would be expected, the differential disappears, with a rate of 46.7 per cent. The total number of recorded HIV-positive cases in the EU is unknown.

These figures are disturbing and are rendered more so by the estimates of increased mobility across national boundaries. The link between AIDS and HIV infection and intravenous drug use is further cause for concern, given the increases in drug misuse. The European institutions perceive AIDS as a 'major scourge which deserves special attention by the Community' and the original Europe Against AIDS programme was therefore extended for a further two years until December 1995. To extend the initiatives taken against AIDS and expand them to cover other communicable diseases, the Commission produced a proposal for a *Community action programme on the prevention of AIDS and certain other communicable diseases in the context of the framework for action in the field of public health* (COM (94) 413 final).This will be described in more detail in Chapter 7, which deals with specific EU programmes.

There is no doubt that the power of national governments to limit the spread of communicable diseases, and especially HIV, is severely limited, most of all in areas of free movement. Many health care professionals would perceive a complementary global approach as potentially more effective, underpinning the efforts of national health agencies and departments and also providing a framework for their operation. The problem with the current European action programme, as far as AIDS is concerned, is that a common framework for

Table 3. Cumulative total of AIDS cases reported among adults/adolescents* in the European Community by 30 June 1994, broken down by country and transmission group**

Country	Homosexual/bisexual males		Drug addicts		Homosexual/bisexual drug addicts		Haemophiliacs/coagulation disorders		Transfusion recipients***		Heterosexual contact		Nosocomial infection		Other/indeterminate		Total
	N	%	N	%	N	%	N	%	N	%	N	%	N	%	N	%	
European Community																	
Belgium	670	42.4	104	6.6	16	1.0	5	0.3	86	5.4	681	43.1	0	0.0	18	1.1	1580
Denmark	1054	72.3	97	6.7	14	1.0	33	2.3	24	1.6	195	13.4	0	0.0	41	2.8	1458
France	14 935	48.4	7317	23.7	462	1.5	379	1.2	1393	4.5	4691	15.2	0	0.0	1653	5.4	30 830
Germany	7859	69.0	1510	13.3	99	0.9	415	3.6	225	2.0	689	6.0	0	0.0	599	5.3	11 396
Greece	498	52.6	40	4.2	9	1.0	63	6.7	45	4.8	100	10.6	0	0.0	191	20.2	946
Ireland	136	34.2	177	44.5	8	2.0	27	6.8	0	0.0	45	11.3	0	0.0	5	1.3	398
Italy	3314	14.6	14 929	65.7	508	2.2	217	1.0	263	1.2	2415	10.6	0	0.0	1074	4.7	22 720
Luxembourg	44	54.3	14	17.3	0	0.0	3	3.7	2	2.5	10	12.3	0	0.0	8	9.9	81
Netherlands	2370	76.0	296	9.5	30	1.0	48	1.5	33	1.1	294	9.4	0	0.0	47	1.5	3118
Portugal	665	34.6	519	27.0	0	0.0	40	2.1	64	3.3	520	27.0	0	0.0	116	6.0	1924
Spain	3899	15.5	16 537	65.8	536	2.1	477	1.9	229	0.9	2016	8.0	0	0.0	1444	5.7	25 138
United Kingdom	6917	74.5	518	5.6	149	1.6	405	4.4	91	1.0	1098	11.8	0	0.0	105	1.1	9283
EC total	42 361	38.9	42 058	38.6	1831	1.7	2112	1.9	2455	2.3	12 754	11.7	0	0.0	5301	4.9	108 872

* Cases aged 13 years or over (46 cases of unknown age could not be classed either as adults/adolescents or as infants).
** Following case reclassification, the figures per transmission group have been modified in certain countries.
*** Includes patients having received transplants or blood products.
Source: *Europe Against AIDS Report*, Com (94) 525 final. Reproduced with the kind permission of the Commission of the European Communities.

tackling it is unlikely to be universally acceptable, given the diverse cultural mores and attitudes of the different EU countries. (The attitudes of the various Member State governments towards drug misuse, as previously described, is an indication of this.) Achievements will therefore inevitably be limited, but if progress is ever to be made on curbing the spread of AIDS it must clearly be on a pan-European, or even international basis.

Common themes and concerns in health service delivery across the European Union

Given the common impact of the various trends affecting health services across Europe (and indeed, much of the developed world) it is not surprising that many services are preoccupied with the same concerns. This is not to say that their operational strategies have been the same; the health services within the various Member States are extremely varied in their structure, organization, funding mechanisms and delivery styles, and have developed their own distinctive strategies for dealing with the problems facing them. Certain themes and concerns are, however, almost universal. Some are explored below.

Primary health care (PHC)

The role of primary health care is reasonably well-established in the EU, with a number of countries having successfully transferred resources into PHC provision. Most governments will continue to shift resources away from acute in-patient care towards primary and community-based provision. Primary care physicians are also likely to take on more responsibility for guiding patients through the health care system and acting as mentors and advisers.

In contrast, the realization of the potential of nurses in the EU as providers of primary health care is hampered by their general lack of involvement in policy-making and decision-making. This is partly due to the poor status of nursing as a profession compared with medicine, and also to the combination of shortages of nurses and a tendency for health care providers to utilize banks of temporary or agency staff, rather than develop nursing staff professionally.

However, PHC is not without its problems, such as uneven geographic availability and distribution, and poor communications between service users and providers, especially in relation to ethnic minorities and immigrant groups. The immensity of the modern body of medical knowledge and the need for almost constant updating is also an issue in primary care. The EU has been directing part of its thrust on the creation of an 'information society' towards easy access to remote sources of information and developmental research via its health sector programmes which are part of the Framework Programmes for Research and Technological Development (for an example, see the case study of the 'Telegastro' project in Chapter 8).

Quality in Europe

International agreements and conventions including the 1950 European Convention for the Protection of Human Rights and Fundamental Freedoms, the Declaration of the Rights of the Patient, adopted in 1981 by the World Medical Association, and more recently, the Declaration on the Promotion of Patients' Rights in Europe (WHO consultation in Amsterdam, 28–30 March 1994) have all been influential in promoting the issue of patients' rights in regard to quality of service.

In the UK, the Patient's Charter has made the issue of quality explicit to the public and helped to create a level of expectation about quality of service in the NHS. Most other EU countries have not attempted to define and communicate the level of quality they aim to achieve, but this does not mean that they are not working to high quality standards. Quality assurance (QA) has become a concern in health care throughout the EU, particularly in relation to patient well-being, customer satisfaction and cost-effectiveness. Some countries, including Belgium, Germany, Italy, the Netherlands, Norway and the UK, have indicated that they intend to integrate quality aspects into future legislation. Considerable research has been directed at QA systems and practice, co-ordinated both at national and international levels. The idea of using techniques common to systems such as total quality management (TQM), which originated in manufacturing industries, has been received with some interest but there are difficulties in transferring such techniques to the health sector on an international or pan-European scale.

One of the most obvious problems is the differences between the national systems, which make collection of data and comparisons of results difficult. Common indicators of quality have been agreed in certain fields such as perinatal and obstetric care, diabetes, and others, and several European databases have been established to focus on agreed common outcomes. These cover areas like diabetes management, orthopaedic surgery and oral health care. (Information is central to any quality system, and there has been a lack of easily available information on EU health systems and indicators. In the future, the Commission's health monitoring programme (due to start in 1997) should make a difference, but is long overdue.)

A user-friendly computer program has been developed by the Organization for Economic Co-operation and Development (OECD), designed to enable hospital managers to monitor their performance against health systems in other countries. The program was produced in response to the widespread demand for factual information on health care internationally. It enables comparisons between 25 health care systems on such aspects as:

- the health status of the population;
- patient care facilities;
- medical staffing;
- expenditure on medical goods and services;
- patterns of hospital delivery.

However, as both citizens and health care professionals become more geographically mobile, difference in practice relating to matters such as consent, access to medical records and legal enforcement of patients' rights will focus attention on quality issues and patient expectation. (A study undertaken on behalf of the WHO Europe (1993), entitled *The Rights of Patients in Europe: a comparative study* by H.J.J. Leenan, J.K.M. Gevers and G. Pinet, addresses these issues in more detail.)

Health care reforms

The various bodies providing combined support for health service users, i.e. the state, the market, the voluntary sector and informal carers, have become more explicitly recognized in most European countries.

Changes are taking place in planning, funding and provision of health services across EU countries and reforms of one type or another have been introduced. These changes have been made in response to national and local needs within the countries concerned and are not in any way an attempt to harmonize health services across the European Union. Health services were diverse before the reforms and they remain diverse after them.

Although there are some countries where reforms appear to be leaning towards convergence, this is probably due to politically motivated, ideologically based factors rather than a desire to create a European health service. The financing of health care is particularly diverse, with countries such as Belgium, France, Germany and Luxembourg supporting health care mainly by social insurance, with delivery in the hands of a mixture of public and private providers, whilst some other countries (e.g. the UK, Denmark, Spain) use finance via direct taxation and mainly public providers. So many European countries are currently reforming their health systems, or have recently done so, that the need for information on the outcomes of health systems and their effectiveness was identified as a priority. The Nuffield Institute for Health, based at the University of Leeds, is leading a project funded under the European Biomedical and Health R&D programme to establish a European Clearing House on Health Outcomes (ECHHO). (Those wishing to read more about health care reforms in European countries should refer to the report entitled *The Future of European Health Care* (1993).)

Cost containment

There are significant differences in the proportion of gross domestic product (GDP) spent on health care throughout the Member States (see Table 4). For example, France spends 9.1 per cent compared with Greece's 5.2 per cent (LSE Health, Occasional Paper No. 2, 1994 by Brian Able-Smith and Elias Mossialos: *Cost Containment and Health Care Reform – a Study of the European Union*). All countries are faced with similar problems which result in massive demands being made on health budgets (expenditure on health has risen in all EU countries with the exception of Sweden). The accelerating demographic changes already described, together with rising expectations of health and technological developments, increasing population mobility both within and across national barriers, the increase of chronic disease and wide-ranging

Table 4.   Total health expenditure

Country	Total expenditure on health		
	% of GDP	Expenditure per capita (ECU)	Total expenditure (MECU)
Belgium	7.9	1273	12 530
Denmark	6.5	1333	6869
France	9.1	1538	87 770
Germany	8.5	1687	108 050
Greece	5.2	288	2964
Ireland	7.3	733	2580
Italy	8.3	1340	77 440
Luxembourg	7.2	1395	528
Netherlands	8.3	1281	19 290
Portugal	6.8	384	3783
Spain	6.7	727	28 370
UK	6.6	939	53 860
EC Median (1991)	7.25	1276	15 910

Source: *The health systems of European Community Member States.* Working Document. The European Parliament Directorate General for Research (1993). Reproduced with kind permission from the Commission of the European Communities.

socio-economic factors, are all creating considerable pressures on national health care systems, and consequently on national governments to increase spending on health.

Different methods have been utilized to contain costs in the various EU countries, and though some have been more successful than others, no long-term, pan-European strategy has been devised as yet. Health promotion and disease prevention are seen as potentially successful long-term measures, along with social measures to reduce the causes of ill-health (such as anti-poverty strategies, stress reduction, etc.) but benefits from these are likely to take a considerable time to be realized. Such activities receive only a tiny amount of funding from health budgets and tend to be severely under-resourced.

Advances in technology, plus increasing longevity, will continue to mop up whatever additional resources are made available. Whilst the debate on rationing of health care is likely to become more intense in the future, and is already a hot political issue in the UK, the benefits of health promotion and education strategies are much more long-term and are therefore not currently perceived as vote winners by any of the British political parties. This is unfortunate, given the potential savings and improvements.

Another key strategy being promoted by the European Commission in implementing European policies is the need to assess the socio-economic impact of new initiatives and developments in order to identify and minimize their negative results – in other words, to ensure that we do not create a whole new set of health problems or establish a climate in which these might thrive. An example of this is the introduction of the information society and the encouragement of widespread use of telematics technology.

Some examples of cost containment measures

The reduction in numbers of hospital beds is a pan-European trend. However, it is clear that this measure will only assist in containing costs if it is based on accurate assessments of declining need, as opposed to the desire to maintain a competitive edge by providers who use the resources released from ward closures to offer a range of other services.

Germany currently has the highest ratio of hospital beds to service users and has introduced a payment system to doctors which encourages the use of day hospitals and daytime surgery. Day hospitals and other daytime facilities, together with low-dependency patient hotels and out-patient facilities, are on the increase and are expected to be part of national government strategies to contain health costs in the EU. Private sector service provision for certain groups, including the elderly, the mentally ill and people with learning disabilities, is also considered to be an effective way of reducing health budgets. In Denmark, this has been speeded up by a process which requires local municipalities to reimburse the county authority, which funds hospital care, for each day an elderly person is kept in hospital waiting for a place in a residential home. Denmark has also developed a dynamic and extensive home nursing service (in direct contrast to most other European countries) which is perceived as more appropriate to the rural nature of much of the country with its lack of large urban conurbations and emphasis on many smaller communities.

Some Member States control either the prices or the profits of the pharmaceutical industries operating within their remit, and all countries have a cost-sharing policy for prescriptions.

All cost-containment strategies are dependent for their success on comprehensive and meaningful data about the health needs of particular populations. Technology now enables rapid information processing and recent IT developments such as telematics have considerable potential for use in the health sector. Unfortunately, the use currently made of IT in the health field across the EU is extremely limited and the sector lags behind most others in its use of information technology. (The European Commission believes that substantial savings and improvements in communication could be achieved by maximizing the potential of IT in health care, and is attempting to encourage this by providing financial incentives via funded programmes.)

According to the study undertaken by Andersen Consulting and Burson-Marsteller, on *The Future of European Health*

Care (1993) (supported by the Hospital Committee of the European Community and the European Association of Hospital Managers), more than 60 per cent of respondents believed that increased competition should be encouraged as a cost containment strategy. Other key findings or forecasts included:

1 Private funding will rise as health care expenditure outstrips economic growth.
2 Citizens will take on more responsibility for their health care needs.
3 Governments will continue to guarantee access and quality whilst controlling costs.
4 The shift to primary/community health care will continue.
5 'Managed' competition will increase.
6 Hospitals will undergo a significant change.
7 Doctors will assume broader responsibilities.
8 The role of the European Community in health care will increase.
9 Information technology will bring significant benefits.

Conclusions

Most policy makers and practitioners agree that a great deal could be achieved by closer collaborative working between Member State health systems and agencies, even at the most basic level – that of information gathering and dissemination. At present there is no standardized detailed description of health care systems within EU Member States which is easily available and accessible to the planner or practitioner, and neither is there a comprehensive information system on health care concerns and practice. Data exists but must be sought in turn from the appropriate organization, and often is unsuitable for purposes of pan-European comparisons because it is not comparing 'like with like'. Information is emerging slowly, as in the case of the studies quoted throughout this book (for example, the Eurocare project), but it needs to be collated and made available to practitioners easily and quickly if it is to be effective in improving patient care.

The whole issue of information availability is crucial to the health care profession and is a major concern. Research and development work, however important and ground-breaking, is of no use if its outcomes are not effectively disseminated. Innovative practices and solutions developed in one region will only produce transferable benefits if the trouble is taken to transfer information about them. Planners and practitioners rarely have the time, resources or inclination to actively search for such information, therefore global authorities must ensure that dissemination is built into national and international budgets and planning. To neglect this would be simply false economy. In addition, the timing of information dissemination is a crucial factor, in order to ensure that research results and improvements and innovations are rapidly made available to health professionals. Quality is a further concern, especially as to accuracy and reliability of information.

The universal change in emphasis from treating the sick to maintaining well-being requires a concerted action plan which involves all the agencies which have a part to play. The task is quite simply to set about managing attitudinal change, not only within the health care professions but for the media, educators, parents and employers, and ultimately the general public. Health education and promotion of healthy lifestyles is the main thrust here, with the aim being to positively promote health rather than react to illness. At its broadest, this concept would emphasize models of well-being and discourage the tendency to project negative images of weakness, vulnerability and sickness in relation to certain groups like the elderly. (Unfortunately, this message is likely to continue to be less than wholeheartedly received by the public, especially in areas where governments appear to be saying one thing and doing another.) This obviously can only be achieved on a pan-European basis, or even on an international scale. Staff development and training for the provision of high quality health services across the EU are similarly in need of more active collaboration and transnational development of the curriculum.

Clearly, these are the principles underlying EU policies, though they neither go far enough nor are adequately funded and disseminated; however, they are a step in the right direction. Worryingly, there has been recent speculation that public health could be an area tagged for 'repatriation' to Member States as a result of the 1996 inter-governmental conference. In early 1995, the *Financial Times* reported that Jacques Delors had been understood to believe that health was an inappropriate area for EU competence and activity, and since then the issue has recurred. Opinions within member states are varied, with the UK traditionally opposing greater powers at EU level in almost any area other than the purely economic. In contrast, the French Minister for Health, Mme Simone Veil, stated that she would support the development of a more far-reaching European health policy and a broader interpretation of Article 129. This would almost certainly require a fully-fledged Directorate General for health (rather than a section of DGV, and a network into other DGs), and a more actively co-ordinated approach to combating disease and health problems, with the capacity to work with the various relevant national and international agencies in order to tackle issues holistically (such as drug and substance misuse).

Pro-European health practitioners, with the interests of the patient at heart, would almost certainly welcome such an extension and perceive nothing but opportunities and benefits arising from it. Those who currently hold the purse-strings and the power in the management of national health care systems, like all builders and holders of empires, are more likely to perceive threats to their 'sovereignty'.

Summary points

1 Health today is at the centre of political and economic crisis and controversy – and a favourite theme for the media and public opinion.
2 Although there is continuing diversity between health systems within the Union, they share a lot in common – particularly rising health costs and the problems to which they relate.
3 The need for a 'level playing field' for the success of the Union, is as urgent in health care as it is in industry and commerce.

4 The mechanisms created by the Union for combining forces in health protection, in areas like cardiovascular disease, cancer, communicable disease and mental health problems, provide an unprecedented opportunity for collaboration on health problems and solutions – particularly when co-ordinated with the efforts of the World Health Organization.

5 Health care measures cannot be self-contained. They have to be reconciled with other political and economic considerations, and are therefore vulnerable to pressures from other quarters. The promotion of healthy lifestyles, for example, is not compatible with some aspects of the Common Agricultural Policy.

6 The ageing population is a European feature particularly challenging to health care systems. One of the Union's sternest tasks is to try and turn round the negative image of the elderly which in itself is exacerbating the problem.

7 Dealing with drug misuse and sexual health – particularly the major scourge of AIDS – are areas where clear advantages can be identified for pan-European action, but ones where differences in national interests and attitudes are dominating and hampering progress.

8 Given the general impact of various trends affecting health services across Europe, many providers are sharing the same preoccupations, although their operational strategies vary. Some common themes and concerns are the role of primary health care, quality assurance, systems reform and cost containment.

9 Most policy makers and practitioners agree that a great deal could be achieved by closer collaborative working, but even at the most basic level of information gathering and dissemination, data is not yet easily transferable or accessible.

10 The principles underlying the Union's approach to health care are laudable. Their implementation is a step in the right direction, but does not go far enough, is inadequately funded, and is limited in impact. Is there also a risk that the inter-governmental conference of 1996 may bring about a retreat from the high tide of Maastricht and the repatriation of public health?

References and further reading

Communication on the framework for action in the field of public health. COM (93) 559 final. Commission of the European Communities.

EUROSTAT. (1993/1). *Rapid Reports, Population and Social Conditions.* EUROSTAT.

EUROSTAT Yearbook '95. (1995). A statistical eye on Europe 1983–1993. EUROSTAT.

The Future of European Health Care. (1993). London: Andersen Consulting.

Health in Europe No. 56. (1994). WHO Europe.

Leenan, H. J. J., Gevers, J. K. M. and Pinet, G. (1993). *The Rights of Patients in Europe: a comparative study.* Kluwer on behalf of WHO Europe.

May, A. (ed.) (1993). *Healthcare in Europe.* Macmillan Magazines.

Report on the integration of health protection requirements in Community Policies. COM (95) 196 final. Commission of the European Communities.

World Health Organization (1992). Proceedings of the first meeting of the Working Party on Health Care Reforms in Europe. Madrid, 23–24. WHO.

7

Freedom of movement – have diploma, will travel?

Aims of this Chapter

In this chapter, we aim to:
- briefly summarize the legislation aimed at facilitating professional mobility;
- consider the current situation with regard to British people;
- identify some of the barriers to free movement;
- explain the measures taken to assist recognition of qualifications across Europe;
- raise some issues about education and training, especially the 'European dimension';
- provide examples of differences in practice and attitude across the EU;
- provide guidance for those wishing to live and work in another Member State, in the form of a personal action checklist.

Movement is of course important not just because it offers the potential to enlarge the careers of health workers and broaden their professional horizons, but primarily, one hopes, because it provides a means of helping to improve the lives of ordinary people throughout the EC.

Sir David Innes Williams, Chairman of the Standards of Excellence Series
(Healthcare Delivery in the European Community, 1992.)

The vision of a frontier-free Europe

The goal of human mobility is one of the four freedoms central to the realization of the European Union, but at present it is far from being achieved. There are relatively few mobile workers, even in professional groups, and the reasons for this are obvious; legal barriers may have been lifted in theory, but there are still many real, practical problems plus the imaginary obstacles which exist inside people's heads.

However, if long-term mobility is still in its infancy, there is now a significant amount of short-term mobility in the form of student and academic visits and exchanges, short-term work placements and the like. This is set to increase further, especially as the new European programme 'Socrates' provides some funding for school-based transnational projects and exchanges.

There has also been an increase in the numbers of people buying property in other Member States in recent years. This has involved relatively small numbers of people and the impact on the host countries (most notably France) has yet to be understood. There is also an established trend of northern Europeans choosing to retire to southern European locations.

All of these people are themselves users of services, including health and social services, and have the right to access these on the same terms as Member State nationals (although those retiring to another country must be financially independent and not a burden on the host economy). This increased mobility on the part of service users (not forgetting tourists), is bound to result in comparisons being made between the services of a host country and the country of origin, and have implications for service providers in due course.

Returning to the issue of professional mobility, which is the focus of this chapter, there is no doubt that the free movement of economically active people is a crucial plank in the construction of the European Union. It is necessary not only to address economic and employment-related problems such as skills shortages between countries, but to ensure the cross-fertilization of ideas and the dissemination of best practice. The real richness of Europe is not deposited in its museums and art galleries but in the living culture, talents and capabilities of its people, but the potential of this will only be fully realized when we are able to work together.

Freedom of movement: the legislative background

In 1957, the Treaty of Rome established certain fundamental principles including the right of European Community citizens to move freely between Member States and to take up paid employment. This, together with other freedoms, went unnoticed by the majority of the population, largely due to lack of information from both European as well as national sources. The necessary measures to ease freedom of movement were only taken after the new impetus of the Single Market programme was introduced to blow the EC out of the doldrums which had becalmed it (as explained in Chapter 2).

The Single European Act re-stated and gave greater clarity to the four freedoms of movement (goods, services, capital and people) and the measures which implemented the Act, via the Single Market programme, finally tackled the legal barriers head-on. European citizens now have the right to live and work anywhere in the EU. However, this does not mean that barriers no longer exist; the legal ones may have been addressed, but there are others which prevent free movement for the mass of the population as effectively as did the Berlin Wall, though less tangibly.

The barriers to mobility

The barriers to mobility throughout Europe appear to outweigh the benefits, at least in people's perceptions if not in reality. The result is that relatively few health care workers have actually been moving freely around Europe, and consequently little information is available on their experiences.

There is no doubt that many barriers do still exist, though they tend not to be physical ones. Studies such as Ness *et al.*, (1993) and Buchan *et al.* (1992) (references provided in the recommended reading section for this chapter) confirm a number of the obvious ones and speculate on some other possibilities.

Insularity

The most significant barriers to mobility are usually those within our own heads. UK citizens demonstrate continually that they simply do not feel themselves to be Europeans, and the British media reinforce this by encouraging a 'them and us' attitude towards the European Union. This is not to say that the other Member States are unanimous in their support and totally uncritical of the EU, but they appear to believe that European unity is a far better option than the alternative. British tabloid headlines along the lines of the famous (or infamous) 'Up yours, Delors!' are usually met with blank astonishment in mainland Europe. Other countries in Europe may also demonstrate these attitudes of insularity to some degree, but it is particularly marked in the UK. (Some Member States have other problems too, including the memory of occupation during wartime.)

The paradox is that this fundamental insularity does not extend to American culture, which we have embraced wholeheartedly and without any negative perceptions (unlike the French, who regard it as a threat to French culture). In fact, we are perhaps less orientated towards Europe in the latter part of the twentieth century than at some other periods in our history.

This tendency to look across the Atlantic rather than the Channel means that relatively few British people are psychologically attuned towards living and working in another European country. Other nationals are more accustomed to crossing borders as a matter of course, because these are frequently artificial boundaries rather than the very real barrier of the sea. (This does not mean that the French feel less French or the Germans less German.)

European initiatives are being taken to address this problem. In 1988, Education ministers meeting within the European Council adopted a Resolution on the European dimension in education, to strengthen the sense of European identity for students as well as increase their knowledge of European issues. This European dimension is only now being introduced to a number of education, training and development programmes in order to prepare people for a pan-European future, rather than a purely national one. In the view of some influential figures, this is a case of 'too little, too late'. For all that, it can only be a welcome development even if it is long overdue.

According to Sir David Innes Williams, 'If Britain is to take a fair share of the multitude of trade and career opportunities which the new Single Market is expected to create, then people here must be prepared to make some effort to get to know and understand the people and societies of their colleague Member States, must begin, in other words, to see themselves as Europeans as well as British'. (Williams, 1992.)

The insularity of the British is also bolstered by a 'Britain knows best' attitude which prevails within a number of sectors including health care. (This belief in our own practice being best is belied by some of the statistics on, for example, cancer treatment.) It also inevitably contributes to the insularity of our strategic planning, as well as our traditional programmes of training and professional preparation and development. 'We can say that there are excuses and exceptions but the fact is that the majority of nurses and doctors are woefully ignorant of the European scene and have only recently become aware of their own ignorance.' (Williams, 1992).

Language

This is probably the greatest and most obvious barrier to free movement, and is the factor which most frequently determines the destination of the migrant. For example, English is widely spoken in many parts of the world and the 'colonies' were for many years the favoured destination of British migrants. The shared language was (often mistakenly) felt to indicate a shared culture and mores, and migrants felt assured of a relatively easy transition to their new society. An unfamiliar language is perhaps the most potent of barriers in the minds of a generally monoglot nation and this is expressed in some of our common sayings and clichés ('It was all Greek to me').

Part of the problem is that foreign languages have been taught and presented within our education system as academic subjects, rather than as a practical means of communication. We have failed to perceive that language skills are essential for personal and professional success in a polyglot world and that has effectively rendered us vulnerable, either confined to the English-speaking world or at the mercy of professional interpreters if we venture beyond our boundaries. If we depend on our professional colleagues' ability to speak English, we can effectively take part in dialogues only at their convenience.

A study undertaken by Ness *et al.* (1993) on mobility of nurses across Europe identified language as the major barrier perceived by the respondents surveyed. Employers will naturally refuse to take on staff who cannot communicate effectively in the host language. Holiday-level fluency in a language is obviously insufficient for professions where there is considerable interaction with patients, often of a highly personal and confidential nature. The study recommends that 'working knowledge of another European language should be encouraged and language skills learned in school should be actively maintained during training'.

All recent European Commission documents on education and training stress the importance of language learning and there is a long-standing commitment to retaining the diversity of European languages, rather than allowing one or two dominant languages to become pre-eminent.

Some countries have programmes of language training in schools which ensure that most of the adult population has a knowledge of at least one other language, and many professionals are fluent in more than one. The Scandinavian countries, together with the Netherlands, Belgium and also Germany are notable examples of this policy.

The danger of allowing this situation to continue in the UK is that it effectively renders our own employment market open to those who have the qualifications and the skills, including fluency in English, to enter it, whilst ensuring that the job markets of the rest of Europe are effectively closed to British professionals. Some companies are beginning to perceive foreign language proficiency as a 'core' skill, and statistics indicate a correlation between language competence and higher income occupations, though in certain countries, notably the Netherlands and Denmark, proficiency in a second language is relatively common. In several EU countries, a foreign language is a compulsory subject at secondary school level, and in certain circumstances pupils are expected to take two languages. English is the most commonly studied of all European languages, with 83 per cent of secondary education students taking it in 1991/2. In contrast, 32 per cent took French, 16 per cent German and only 9 per cent Spanish, despite the fact that some of the world's Spanish-speaking countries are experiencing particularly rapid economic growth. (*Key data on education in the European Union, 1994,* 1995.)

Social and economic barriers

Even moving to find work *within* one's own Member State can be an emotional wrench for many people, who experience a culture shock in moving from, say, Merseyside to London. This is particularly true for those accustomed to the support of extended family groups and friends of long standing. Familiarity with the customs and practices of an area, in the workplace as well as in one's home life, is for many an essential component of their personal and professional confidence. To begin again in an unfamiliar country, where everything must be learned from scratch, can be a terrifying prospect and one which is quite literally unthinkable to many individuals who have firm roots in one place.

An additional consideration is the issue of social and welfare support, which may differ greatly in the 'new' country. Those with dependants, whether children or the elderly, will be influenced by the level of support and by the types of facilities and amenities available to them at their proposed destination. Those people considering a permanent move will need to consider pension and social security arrangements. Older people who have paid considerable pension contributions already will need to decide whether they can afford to retire in their new country and live off pension payments in sterling, given the fluctuations of the exchange rate.

There are, of course, others who regard making such a move as an exciting, invigorating challenge and an opportunity to build a new life.

Occupational mismatches

One of the real, practical difficulties facing some workers is that their jobs do not automatically translate across the borders of one country to another. Some occupations which have developed out of the culture and economic and social context of one country may simply not exist in another, or may be so different as to be unrecognizable. (Some examples are provided later in the chapter.)

Recognition of qualifications and professional competence

This remains a barrier for many people who might wish to work in another EU country, although considerable efforts have been made by the European Commission to address the issue. It will be explored more thoroughly in the following section, which considers the issue of recognition of professional competence and qualification in some detail.

Professional qualifications and their acceptance across the EU

In the early days of the EEC, professionals wishing to work in another Member State simply had to re-qualify in order to take up a post, as there was no mechanism or approved pathway to recognition of professional qualifications. The European Commission, perceiving that this was a real barrier to mobility, attempted to set in train a process for dealing with the issue.

The initial approach to freedom of movement for professional workers was to carry out an exercise to scrutinize each profession in turn and to agree a basis for mutual recognition, which would be implemented via a specific European directive. This 'sectoral approach' was undertaken by carefully examining the education and training requirements and the professional responsibilities of the group concerned in an attempt to 'harmonize' requirements across Europe. It was a complex and difficult task, partly because professional groups such as architects had different education and training programmes in different countries and even different responsibilities and approaches to their jobs, and partly because there was a great deal of detailed work to be done on each professional group. (The work on the directive on professional recognition for architects was said to have taken 17 years.) The process was extremely laborious and inflexible, and eventually was abandoned altogether.

This initial attempt at smoothing the way for professional workers resulted in a number of sectoral directives, including those dealing with GPs, nurses (general care), midwives, veterinary surgeons, dentists and pharmacists.

The General System Directive

The European Commission then proposed a bolder and more sweeping approach to professional qualifications. The attempt at harmonization having failed, the Commission proposed that qualifications requiring at least three years of higher education and relating to regulated professions should be subject to 'mutual recognition'. This proposal was made in a Directive (89/48/EEC) agreed by the Council of Ministers in December 1988, with an implementation date of 4 January 1991. The UK actually implemented it via regulations which came into effect on 17 April 1991, three months late, but was only the second Member State to do so (Ireland being the only one to meet the deadline).

The position created by the General System Directive, as it was known, was much simpler than the harmonization approach. However, it only applied to *regulated* professions, and the difficulty was that not all the same professions are regulated in every Member State. From 1993, the Directive also applied to the EFTA (European Free Trade Area) countries as well.

The Directive recognized that there could be significant differences between the education and training and the activities of the same professional group in different Member States, and created safeguards in order to protect professional standards. The first of these is concerned with differences in the length of professional education and training; if professionals wish to practise in a country where the training period is longer than that they have themselves undertaken, they may be required to produce evidence of up to four years' professional experience in order to establish their competence. The second safeguard is concerned with the content of professional education and training provision, and where this differs significantly, professionals may be required to take an aptitude test or a period of supervised professional practice ('the adaptation period') which would be assessed in order to establish professional competence.

The professionals themselves would normally decide which of these to choose, except in cases where a precise knowledge of national law is required by the profession concerned; in such cases, the Member State would decide which of the safeguards to apply. However, professionals cannot be asked to undertake both safeguards or be re-tested, or for that matter, be required to re-qualify in areas already covered by their professional training.

How it works in practice

The Directive ensures that all professionals to whom its provisions apply have a legal right to have their qualifications recognized and to subsequently practise in another European Member State. In order to do this they must apply to the relevant 'designated authority' for recognition, providing evidence of their qualifications and experience as necessary. (An example of how this works in practice is given later in this chapter, in the account provided by a Dutch psychologist working in the UK.) The designated authority, which must respond within four months, can reject the application but must have significant grounds for doing so, and the applicant has the right of appeal to a national court or other body.

Otherwise the designated authority must either accept the application and process it accordingly, or invoke one of the safeguards already described.

The UK situation

The UK government has allocated responsibility for ensuring the correct application of the Directive to the Department of Trade and Industry. However, whilst the DTI has produced an advisory booklet on mutual recognition, *The Single Market – Europe Open for Professions* (DTI and Central Office of Information, 1992), and is willing to give general advice, it regards the matter as one principally for the designated authorities. The DTI booklet lists the professions covered by the Directive in the UK and the relevant designated authorities.

Some problems associated with the General System approach

Although the system of mutual recognition was introduced primarily to facilitate free movement of professionals, it has produced some problems of its own. The intention was to enable individual professions to achieve harmonization at their own pace, using the mutual recognition mechanism as a tool for doing so. However, the momentum for this now appears to have been lost, and some professional groups, including health care professionals, are worried about the feasibility of maintaining high standards within a system based on mutual recognition of qualifications.

The Directive makes provision for individuals to make up for any shortcomings in their education and training but in reality the means of doing so have proved expensive and difficult to arrange, and therefore unpopular. Employing organizations are naturally reluctant to offer posts to applicants who need to undertake periods of supervision before they can be allowed to practise, and the assessment system itself obviously carries a cost.

Information on registrations of professionals across Member State boundaries is limited, but the process of registration itself can be complex and bureaucratic (Ness *et al.* 1993). However, this could be partly due to the fact that many designated authorities lack experience of the process, as a result of so few applications being made to them.

As far as the nursing profession is concerned, some nurses are covered by sectoral directives whilst others (psychiatric nurses for example) are covered by the General System Directive. The UKCC and the RCN are aware of the problems created by this situation, together with those outlined above, and are keen to support those experiencing difficulties (Pritchard and Wallace, 1994: 211–15).

A Second General System Directive (Council Directive 92/51/EEC) of 18 June 1992 supplemented the original General System Directive and specifically mentioned the UK system of National Vocational Qualifications (NVQs) and Scottish Vocational Qualifications (SVQs).

Other approaches

Workers wishing to exercise their right to free movement will naturally wish to ensure that their qualifications, wherever possible, meet the legal or regulatory requirements laid down for their profession in their country of destination. But the obstacles to professional mobility are not all legal ones: there are many non-regulated professions which do not benefit from the arrangements described above. Many staff working within the health and welfare sector will not be covered by the directives described above, which apply mainly to those in narrowly defined 'professional' groups. Only those people within the professions covered by specific directives or by the General System Directives will have the right to recognition of their qualifications, which will 'oil the wheels' and assist their professional mobility as workers. Those outside will have to rely on other means, including many of the skilled technicians and support staff so essential to the smooth running of health systems.

More informal approaches have been tried to facilitate free movement in these cases, and are based upon the idea that information on occupations and vocational training should be made more easily available so that employers and workers are not simply left to their own devices.

Comparability of vocational training

A Council Resolution of 16 July 1985 (85/638/EEC) proposed the establishment of a system for the comparability of vocational training qualifications across the European Community. The work was carried out by groups of experts from the Member States, and co-ordinated by CEDEFOP, the European Centre for Vocational Training. They concentrated on comparing the jobs and training of workers across a range of selected occupational areas. The areas covered did not include health care but the basic principle, if found to be successful, could have been applied to any occupational area.

The approach was to select certain jobs within occupational groupings and to reach agreement on common tasks performed by workers within that occupation, to arrive at a 'Euro Job Description'. Qualifications relating to the specified job were noted and the information was presented in tabulated form. However, the approach was eventually abandoned as being too time-consuming and inflexible, especially as new technological developments affected the nature and content of jobs. (The information on comparability is still available for employers and workers who wish to access it, via the Comparability Coordinator based at the (former) Department of Employment at Moorfoot, Sheffield – see the Resource section at the end of this book.)

Transparency of qualification

The Council of Ministers adopted a Resolution in December 1992 (93/C 49/01) which expressed their doubts about the usefulness of the comparability approach and stated the need for 'new directions' towards achieving transparency of qualifications. The Resolution also acknowledged the need to recognize the skills and knowledge acquired by workers outside of formal study and qualifications, as well as the qualifications themselves.

Two key objectives were identified: 'Enabling individuals who so wish to present their occupational qualifications, education and work experience clearly and effectively to potential employers throughout the Community'; and 'Helping employers to have easy access to clear descriptions of qualifications and relevant professional experience in order to establish the relevance of the skills of job applicants from other Member States to jobs on offer'.

This focused firmly upon the need to find a definitive or at least commonly acceptable method of communicating information about a worker's competence in a form understandable and accessible to employers. Within national systems, most employers are familiar with the commonly-accepted qualifications or levels of experience thought appropriate to a job. Once outside the national boundaries, though, these have little or no meaning, and clearly it is impossible to expect every employer to carry out an in-depth interview simply to find out what an applicant is familiar with. Some mechanisms must be available to both employer and employee to facilitate the process.

An example – the portfolio approach

Various developmental projects resulted from the 1992 Transparency Resolution. One of them was the European Portfolio Project, which explored ways of developing an individual portfolio for each worker which could act as a European 'passport' to employment. The underlying thesis for the project was that recruiters and potential employers need to know what a job applicant has learned or is able to do, and the job seekers themselves need to know how to present information in support of their applications in an easily understandable way.

Information about individuals, including a brief summary of their qualifications and achievements gained not only via education and training but in their working lives, could be contained within an 'individual portfolio' under a common format of headings relevant to prospective employers. Use of the portfolio would be voluntary, but if it became sufficiently widespread it would be easily recognized by employers and provide a simple means of communicating information about people wishing to work outside their own 'home' state.

Work on the initial stages of the Portfolio Project was between November 1993 and February 1995, with a UK organization, NCVQ (the National Council for Vocational Qualifications), being the main contractor, and work being carried out across all of the (then) 12 Member States.

The project's findings were that most employers and job-seekers involved welcomed the format of the portfolio, though employers generally wished to retain their own application forms and use portfolios as a supplement to their documentation rather then a replacement for it. The term 'portfolio' was not widely liked or understood and more work needed to be undertaken on the kind of information required by employers. The project report also recommended that development of portfolios needed to be part of a package of measures including more information on national systems of education, training and qualifications, to help employers better understand the information in portfolios. There should also be networks of national experts and ways of checking the accuracy of information provided by applicants.

Advantages of personal portfolios

Portfolios have been used for some time now in various sectors as a means of identifying skills and competences achieved within education and training programmes, at the workplace and in other areas of a person's experience (e.g. via voluntary work). They are also used in the Accreditation of Prior Learning (APL), though this is not a familiar concept in most EU countries outside the UK. The portfolio approach has appeal for health care professionals and other groups working with people because it is a flexible and highly individual means of recording a variety of skills and competences, many of them interpersonal and outside the scope of formal examinations or qualifications. More people who have become familiar with the concept are now maintaining personal portfolios which often include information such as testimonials and references from past employers or line managers, job descriptions and specifications as well as the more usual records of achievement such as certificates and diplomas.

The debate continues...

Post-Maastricht, there was little evidence that the General System Directives had significantly increased professional mobility. The European Commission, conscious of this and concerned that the obstacles to free movement of professionals remained, issued a *Communication on recognition of qualifications for academic and professional purposes* (COM (94) 596 final) in December 1994. It was intended to stimulate debate on how best to co-ordinate recognition of qualification, and identified four 'paths' to follow 'in order to develop the synergies between the different types of recognition of qualifications'. These are intended to be mutually supportive and consist of four broad mechanisms:

- information;
- creation of academic and professional networks;
- joint adaptation of courses;
- evaluation of quality.

One likely outcome is a third directive on recognition of qualifications, which would update and streamline the previous legislation, clarifying issues and simplifying procedures.

Some further 'mobility' issues

Education and training for a mobile workforce – 'Europeanizing' the curriculum

Demographic changes, especially the ageing of the population, will inevitably result in additional strains upon the health and welfare systems of all European states. The need for a well-educated, highly motivated and adaptable workforce has been stated frequently by both 'partners in industry' (i.e. management and unions), but the need for such a workforce to have the transferable skills to enable them to operate across the European Union has yet to be widely articulated, let alone strategically tackled. The European Commission and Parliament have both reiterated their commitment to such a goal, but many national institutions and organizations responsible for professional education and training are not demonstrating the same zeal for Europeanizing the curriculum. Some are doing so, however, though often on the basis of experimental or prototype courses or modules. Rob Sykes, of the School of Health and Community Studies at Sheffield Hallam University, has been involved in 'Europeanizing' the curriculum there, and writes ...

'**The Context**: In 1994, the School gained support under the Government's ENTERPRISE scheme for the development of a Level 3 (i.e. third-year undergraduate) study unit in its BA Applied Social Studies programme, titled *European Awareness: Employment Skills.*

The Problem: to design a Level 3 study unit which:

- is academically relevant, interesting and challenging to third-year social sciences and similar students;
- accesses up-to-date material in a simple and effective way to support students' independent study and broader learning skills;
- develops students' employment and other transferable skills;
- can also be accessed by ERASMUS students coming to or going from Sheffield Hallam University;
- does all the above in an innovative and flexible way with the use of new technologies etc. so as to maximise accessibility and 'openness' for both home and 'foreign' students;
- and, most importantly, the unit should give students a 'feel' for current developments and the character of 'Europe' which both enthuses and is an enabling influence.

Towards a Solution: two questions were the starting point

1 What is the current level of 'European awareness' and what are the interests of students and staff in 'Europe'?
2 What written and other materials exist to support student learning and skills development in 'European awareness'?

A questionnaire administered to social science students and to all staff in the School provided vital curriculum design information, including:

- 53% of students felt 'under-informed' about European issues;
- 93% of students felt that there should be an increased emphasis in their studies in gaining an awareness of Europe;
- 78% of students said they would be interested in taking a European awareness unit in their study programme;

- students were most interested in studying European social and economic features, European politics and history, European Union institutions and policies and European languages;
- teaching staff identified the following topics as important: European social and economic features, European languages and EU institutions and policies.

A search of literature and other sources revealed a burgeoning number of books on various aspects of Europe, especially the European Union. In addition, a number of CD-ROM and Internet-based materials were found which offered different and exciting opportunities for information-gathering, learning and assessment. It was decided at an early stage to use the facilities offered by these new technologies to support a multimedia approach to the new unit.

Next, ideas for the new unit were discussed with partners in the main ERASMUS inter-university co-operation programme (ICP) to which the School belongs, and a bid was made to the ERASMUS programme to support the development of a European Awareness unit for the ICP which would be accessible to all the students in each participating institution. In May 1995, this bid was approved and the unit originally developed is likely to be adapted and made available to students in all 10 participating European colleges and universities in the ICP. This is a vital feature of the joint curriculum development because, as both the various universities and the European Commission now recognise, 'Europeanising the curriculum' must take account of the fact that the great majority of students will not be taking part in study exchanges. Thus any European awareness input must focus as much on the 'immobile' students as the 'mobile' ones. SOCRATES, the successor programme to ERASMUS, recognises this as a central feature of its strategy. In this context, the use of open and distance learning technologies, including computer and video conferencing, e-mail and remote access to networked databases and other information sources is of prime significance.

The current position and future developments

A unit entitled *Europe and the European Union: Economy, Society and Politics* has been developed. After piloting and further development, this unit will be offered both as a Level 3 undergraduate and as a Level M postgraduate unit. Some of its features are:

- a flexible structure and delivery pattern, with students taking a half module based upon directed reading and information gathering, collation and seminars, and a half module based on a project;
- use of a wide range of recently-published books and articles plus use of CD-ROMs and the Internet;

- coverage of both general socio-economic and political features of Europe and of European Union structure and policies;
- skills development in both individual and group-based study environments.

Work on the project revealed that graded provision of European Awareness units from Level 1 undergraduate through to Postgraduate level across the University would be possible using the model we have developed. We hope that these units can be developed and also that identified CD-ROM material will be made available to all students via the University network.

In the near future, the University is likely to seek recognition from the European Commission as a European Study Centre. Meanwhile, a Community Wide Information System based upon the University's own computer networks, plus the Internet, is being rapidly developed to improve access to a range of facilities for staff and students.

Summing up – the project has successfully developed a range of materials and study/learning methods which open up a wealth of possibilities for greater awareness and understanding of Europe for both students and staff. These can be easily adapted to a variety of levels and courses. The question remains, however, as to whether the course designers, professional validation bodies and academic departments at this and other universities see incorporation of such European material as a central part of their curricula. Until they do, and make moves positively to encourage its incorporation into courses, British students are likely on the whole to remain relatively uninformed about Europe and disadvantaged in the increasingly competitive European labour markets.'

Rob Sykes, School of Health and Community Studies, Sheffield Hallam University

The need for a flexible, professionally competent and responsive health workforce, with its training programmes and professional consciousness placed firmly within a European context, is the underpinning conviction behind this book. Education and training at pre-service level plays a crucial part in this but continuous staff development within different professions is a key element in achieving competence. It also ensures that practising professionals within the various health care sectors are in touch with those developing both the pre-service and staff development curricula by virtue of undertaking ongoing professional training. (The emphasis now being placed on lifelong learning both at national and international levels, is a welcome development, as is the designation of 1996 as 'European Year of Lifelong Learning'.)

Staff development for a European labour market

In 1991, a workshop was organized by the European Healthcare Management Association on behalf of the European Foundation for the Improvement of Living and Working Conditions (and the conclusions were subsequently published as the discussion document *The Health Sector in the European Community – 1992 and Beyond,* 1991). At the workshop, the question of future health care worker preparation was discussed, and there was general agreement that all health care workers and specifically those in public health and health care management would need the skills and breadth of vision to operate on a broader canvas. This would include knowledge of conditions across Europe, including an awareness of major developments, an understanding of how health, social and environmental services are organized and how socio-cultural differences contribute to different experiences of health and health care.

Since 1991 the professional and regulatory bodies have done relatively little to address these concerns and education and training programmes continue to focus primarily, if not solely, on UK health issues and priorities. Any progress made has tended to be in the pre-service sector, and that has usually been initiated within the delivering institution itself, where staff teaching on full- and part-time courses are taking the lead on Europeanizing their curricula and encouraging students to undertake exchanges and study visits to other countries. The Europeanizing of in-service training and staff development and professional networking is well behind. Although the 1992 discussion paper identified that 'the challenge for international bodies, but especially for the professional groups, is to develop fora for contact at a European level', this has only occurred in rare cases. For example, the profession of Occupational Therapy, though a relatively new occupation, has a good record of international liaison via bodies such as the World

Federation of Occupational Therapists (WFOT). In fact, in some cases WFOT is fulfilling a regulatory function: in order to register and practise in certain countries it is necessary to have trained at a WFOT-recognized training centre.

Veterinary surgeons also have a history of pan-European co-operation, partly due to mechanisms established when preparing the Sectoral Directive on harmonization of veterinary qualifications which was issued in 1978 and entered into force in 1980. Transnational activity within the profession continues and the relatively small numbers of institutions delivering training facilitates this. The EC Advisory Committee on Veterinary Training undertook comparisons of training across Member States in order to ensure a reasonably similar core curriculum. This was achieved by site visits, with the aim of visiting all of the 40 veterinary schools every 7–10 years. This kind of exercise would clearly be impossible to apply to professions with larger numbers of training centres but a modified approach could be adopted (e.g. sampling) which would still produce benefit.

In terms of a drive towards curriculum development to integrate the European dimension, there are some positive signs which suggest that change is on the way. The nursing profession's new curriculum guidelines for pre-registration nursing and midwifery, launched in December 1994 under the title of *Creating Lifelong Learners: Partnerships for Care* (ENB), makes reference to the European directives and the nursing curriculum guidelines also refer to the incorporation of a European and international dimension. In the 1995/6 Operational Objectives of the English National Board for Nursing, Midwifery and Health Visiting, the Board states that one of its objectives is: 'To consolidate links with organisations within the European Union with responsibility for the provision and development of nursing and midwifery to facilitate the sharing of good practice' (provided by the ENB in personal correspondence to the authors). The Board has now consolidated links with other organizations within the EU and the information gathered is being used to inform policy development.

The long-awaited document on *Standards for educational experience outside the United Kingdom for students undertaking*

National Board approved programmes leading to registration on the Council register was issued in January 1995 (and is reproduced as Appendix 2 of this chapter). These guidelines should encourage those responsible for nurse education to build into their programmes periods of study and exchange with other Member States. Perhaps other professional groups may be inspired by this example and produce similar guidelines.

Despite the occasional exception, and as already indicated, much of the impetus in curriculum development has come from the field and has emerged from the first hand experience of health care professionals. An interesting example is provided below by Chris Bumstead of an experience gained via the HOPE Exchange Programme and its results:

'The HOPE Exchange Programme was established fifteen years ago as an opportunity for young healthcare administrators to experience at first hand the organisation of healthcare institutions across Europe. It was, and still is, organised under the direction of the Hospitals Committee of the EU but has, with the evolving nature of health management, attracted participants from a broad field, including clinicians, and now offers the opportunity for a more in-depth study of particular areas of interest.

When I took part in the programme in 1992 I was based at a large psychiatric hospital in the Netherlands, which was in the process of moving home to its catchment area in Rotterdam and developing community-based services. My main interest was to study community mental health day facilities. For me, this was a very valuable experience because it enabled me to broaden my vision of healthcare possibilities and learn about good practice, particularly about patient/client empowerment. It is not always possible to transfer ideas and systems directly across national boundaries due to social, cultural and political differences but an awareness of the different approaches to a common problem can be of real help in guiding the process of planning and decision making. It is also an enhancement to professional expertise.

I first heard about the programme by accident, via my mentor during a Health Services Management Certificate course (IHSM/OU). This ad hoc approach to recruitment for the programme still continues and requires some attention. There is also the problem that the programme is an individualised experience which has no formal follow-up which could continue the exchange and assist networking across Europe. To this end, the European Young Health Managers' Association

(EYHMA) was established five years ago by former HOPE exchange participants and now has affiliated members' associations in fourteen countries. This year (1995) I established the Network of European Health Managers (NEHM) as the UK affiliate to EYHMA, and at a recent meeting of the latter in Madrid, it was agreed that a stronger working relationship should be created between the various national Young Health Managers' Associations via small working groups and by developing a common database to encourage networking on topics of interest and concern. A current topic is the debate on 'choices in healthcare and patients' rights'.

Both the HOPE Exchange programme and the EYHMA operate on shoestring budgets but are a valuable vehicle for generating trans-European co-operation in healthcare and the development of common principles of good practice.'

Chris Bumstead, Director of Therapies, Pathfinder Mental Health Services NHS Trust, London, and Chair of the Network of European Health Managers

Generally speaking, professional networking and collaboration on curriculum development has not been the norm to date. However, where collaborative work has been carried out, initiated or encouraged by some means such as funding, it has borne valuable fruit. For example, the *Europe Against Cancer* programme, begun in 1986 and funded by the EU, has produced a number of useful outcomes. As a response to the programme, the EC Advisory Committee on the Training in Nursing set up a Working Group to look at the ways in which cancer care was being taught to nurses in the Member States, both at basic and post-basic level of training, which resulted in a core curriculum for a European post-basic cancer care nursing course. Implementation of the course across the Member States is not without its difficulties but the model could usefully serve as an exemplar for other specialist spheres of practice.

Medical tourism

The use of health care facilities in one country by citizens of another country is likely to increase. This may result from a patient's own decision, referral by a doctor, action by providers to attract patients from other countries, and action by insurers/sick funds/purchasers to buy services from providers in other countries. Any or all of these decisions may be motivated by quality and/or cost considerations. One possibility is that multinational providers will concentrate some of their services in low cost, low wage countries ... The result could be an increased flow of patients to southern States. It is more likely, however, that there will be a flow of patients in the opposite direction to 'centres of excellence' in the centre of the Community. There is already some evidence of the development of an international market for highly specialised services such as transplants.

The Health Sector in the European Community – 1992 and Beyond, 1991

This concept of 'medical tourism', albeit more likely between countries with close linkages via borders and languages, cannot be ignored and should be taken into consideration when organizations are undertaking their strategic planning.

An increase in medical tourism has wide-ranging implications for health staff, not only in terms of education and training needs but in terms of attitudinal and cultural perception. The health care worker of the future must have the ability to care for individuals from a wide range of cultural backgrounds and national groups. Communications skills (not merely a facility in another language) and cultural awareness will be especially important in such a context. Health care professionals have frequently been the subject of criticism for insensitive treatment of patients, including failure to listen effectively or encourage patients to articulate their needs, and the tendency to patronize. These are common human failings but their effect is magnified within health care settings, where the professional is in a position of authority and the patient usually feels extremely vulnerable and lacking in confidence.

Strategic planning and information provision

The complexity of European health workforce planning has been a neglected issue until relatively recently. The broader human resource issues such as skill mix, volume, cost and conditions may have been considered within national boundaries, but there is little evidence of strategic thinking being done within a European context, even for something as fundamental as supply and demand for staff, a recognized and much-discussed area of concern.

Part of the problem is lack of quality information which is easily available to the staff on the ground. The need to engage in pan-European health research and developmental work is becoming more obvious, and transnational activity, including staff exchanges, is increasing. At present, though, information on both developmental activities and health care systems and staffing is held by a variety of different organizations and there is no centralized European source of health-related information. Even information on the health-related projects and developmental work funded directly by the European Union is not readily available, despite the European Commission's commitment to openness and accessibility of information. One obstacle is lack of resources; in the case of research and development projects, for instance, funding is seen to be most appropriately spent on the project work itself and only a small proportion of overall budgets has traditionally been allocated to dissemination of results and outcomes. This is now being addressed by the Commission, but on a limited scale, and largely amongst and between the various clusters of programmes providing funding for programmes – indeed, dissemination between the cognoscenti, in a sense. Much extremely interesting and valuable work is never cascaded down to health care practitioners in the field, though professional updating is possibly more important in the health and welfare sector than any other.

Problems of supply and demand in the health professions

In 1989, a meeting was held in Paris of representatives of EC Community health ministries. The aim was to compare health service staffing situations in different Member States, analyse the problems and identify solutions. The main issues were found to be the over-supply of medical doctors and the shortages of nursing staff existing in most EC countries.

A year later, the Council of Europe's Fourth Conference of European health ministers in Nicosia took as its theme 'Health Manpower: Changes and Challenges'. Yet despite this recognition of staffing as a major issue, little detailed work appears to have been done in terms of analyses and comparisons of professional practice and workloads between European health professionals, even amongst the largest groups like nurses and doctors.

Only recently has the issue been tackled, with a study conducted for the Hospital Committee of the European Community on *Manpower Problems in the Nursing/Midwifery Professions in the EC* (Versieck, Bouten and Pacolet, 1995). The summary and policy conclusions of this report make interesting reading. The report states that the UK has about 12 nurses per 1000 people, compared with 10 per 1000 in Germany, Belgium, Luxembourg and Denmark, and even lower ratios in France and Portugal. The point is made that a shortage of nurses in any one nation of the EU is less likely to be caused by a drop in the supply of trained staff as an increase in demand.

Other data which is currently available seems to indicate that ratios of population to various types of health staff vary considerably between different European countries and that there is little evidence of a common approach to determining levels of demand or utilization of staff. Certain professions do not exist in the same form in some Member States, and there are considerable differences in expectations of professional knowledge and practice. (For example, anyone finding an unfamiliar form of fungi in France would immediately take it to the nearest pharmacy for identification and advice on whether or not it was edible, and possibly receive additional guidance on its preparation for the table! A British high-street chemist would almost certainly be nonplussed by such a request.) No strategic planning in relation to supply and demand of health care staffing is taking place at European level, and mobility is largely the result of personal preferences and individual enterprise (as in the case of the Dutch psychologist whose account of working in the UK appears later in this chapter).

Another problem common throughout Europe is the lack of strategic regulation of intake of students on many health or medical courses relative to need – a problem not confined to the health sector alone. In the UK at present, funding arrangements for further and higher education actually encourage recruitment of students on to courses in order that institutions can meet their recruitment and growth targets, regardless of whether those in training are likely to find jobs at the end of their courses.

Differences in role and status

There are, as might be expected, differences in professional practice and in status between the various groups of health care professionals across the EU. Professional autonomy is affected by factors such as legal and governing body requirements and by codes of practice which differ throughout the EU, and in some cases have yet to be formulated, and the professions which are regulated in one country may not be in another. Consequently the various professional groups are in different stages of development and regulation, and those which lack a national professional identity suffer from associated problems such as lack of influence, low pay, poor conditions of employment and inadequate education and training provision. Trends aimed at cost reductions are having an effect; for example, nursing unions in Denmark are pressing for the employment of more highly qualified personnel whilst the government is considering increasing the numbers of less qualified 'carers'.

Professional autonomy is also a crucial factor in the smooth running of multi-disciplinary health care provision, which itself is in the early stages of development in some countries of the EU. In some cases, the role of one professional group may be affected by under or over supply of another; for example, where there is an over supply of doctors, the role of the midwife may be reduced to that of doctor's assistant. In other cases, geographical factors can affect roles so that nurses with a peripatetic role in rural areas may enjoy increased professional autonomy and status. Certain groups of 'newer' professions are particularly affected by anomalies: in the case of occupational therapists, for instance, private practice is not allowed in Denmark, and in France is restricted to that prescribed by a doctor (Health Care Delivery in the European Community, Standards of Excellence series, 1992). A German Director of Nursing has claimed that British and Irish nurses were reluctant to undertake what they saw as menial tasks, such as emptying urine bottles and refilling laundry carts, though their German colleagues accepted such aspects of the nursing role as part of patient care.

Certain types of work undertaken by radiographers in the UK (e.g. ultrasound) would be the responsibility of doctors in most other Member States. Nurses in France tend to be more technically orientated than in the UK, undertaking electro-cardiographs and taking blood specimens as a matter of course. Such examples serve to illustrate the differences in roles and responsibilities, which have often developed from custom and practice, yet can have a profound effect upon status and consequently professional standing and salary levels.

Even professions which appear to be very similar, in neighbouring countries, will be affected by the health service culture in which they are embedded, as well as the wider culture of the country itself. Only those few health care professionals who have actually experienced working in another country can really appreciate the differences which exist, and the attitudinal adjustments necessary to enable someone rooted in one health care culture to operate successfully in another. One of these is Robin Paijmans, a psychologist from the Netherlands who writes below about his experiences as 'a Dutchman in the UK':

'I completed my Masters' degree in Clinical, Health and Cross-Cultural psychology in the Netherlands in 1991. This is called a "Doctorandus"; the name indicates that you have gained the right to proceed to a PhD (unlike in Britain, where you can do this upon obtaining the Bachelors' degree). Subsequently, I was confronted with the unfortunate situation of a surplus of psychologists in the Netherlands (actually, there is really a shortage, but there are more than the Health Service can afford to employ). It is very hard to obtain even a one-year contract, which means that as soon as you have taken up employment you have to start looking for another post. Having scanned for possible job prospects whilst still at University, I was aware of the chronic shortage of clinical psychologists in Britain.

Working in Britain seemed like an obvious possibility to me also because I had visited the country several times and knew it fairly well (or so I naively thought; I have since found out that actually living and working here is quite different from a three-week holiday in Norfolk or a weekend spent shopping in London). I am quite fluent in the English language, like so many Dutch people, because no-one else in the world can be bothered to speak ours. This is, by the way, no minor consideration in a profession that very much involves communicating with people! And having taken part in an Erasmus student exchange programme to Germany and a Health Psychology course in Rome, I had become used to the idea of seeing the whole of Europe as a job market, especially since 1992 and the Single Market was coming up.

The first thing I did was to talk to British clinical psychologists and psychology students to get an idea of the situation abroad (a useful tip: visit European conferences, meet interesting people and ask many questions). I learned that my first step should be to approach the British Psychological Society, which maintains professional standards and keeps a list of qualified and approved psychologists. Clinical psychologists from abroad wanting to work in the NHS have to obtain from the BPS a Statement of Equivalence, stating that their training is equivalent to that of an approved British Clinical Psychologist. A comparable society exists in the Netherlands, called the NIP (the Netherlands Institute for Psychologists).

For those who think that the European Community means that qualifications are accepted easily across national borders – forget it. What it means for clinical psychologists is that the BPS will provide a conclusive evaluation of your qualifications within four months. This can be a rather complex and abstruse process. You are sent a considerable amount of information to make sense of, together with forms to complete and requests for details about your study curriculum, training, research, etc. (with translations to be provided in English, of course), as well as copies of your degrees and two references. The BPS then judges how far this compares in depth and content to the British training, and decides if, and what, additional experience should be acquired. The BPS benchmark is very thorough and serves to safeguard standards of practice. It involves experience with adult, elderly, learning disabled and child populations, whereas my Dutch training mainly focused on adult mental health. As a result, I was required to gain some additional clinical experience which I am currently doing with my present employer, in return for my full services once I have obtained my Statement of Equivalence.

I have often been asked about my impressions of working in the UK. Not an easy question! The British NHS was the first of its kind on its inception in 1948. It was an ambitious project and served as an example for many other European countries. As a consequence, the Dutch Health Service is in some ways similar to the British NHS, and is now facing similar problems in terms of the increasing cost of more sophisticated medical technology and better health care for a growing population, though this is to some extent attenuated by virtue of higher national health insurance rates.

There has always been tension in the NHS between its idealistic aim of health care for all, irrespective of status or income, and the reality of limited financial resources to meet such standards. The aim of the formation of NHS trusts, as I understand it, was to reorganise health care into a more effective and cost-efficient service. It constitutes a very different approach to that of the Dutch Health Service and it took some time for me to understand how it works. (Imagine my relief when I discovered I was not the only one to be confused!) Nevertheless, I am not convinced that the NHS can be run like a commercial market of service providers competing for purchasers. Competition reduces the selling price of a service or product, but not its cost. The reduction is in the profit margin (hopefully compensated for by increased demand). But the NHS is a people's service, not a profit-making organisation; any reduction in price will force a reduction in the cost of the service itself. Initially this may encourage efficiency but soon it leads to cutting corners and a reduction in quality.

The NHS here also seems to be much more of a theatre of political forces than in the Netherlands. This is perhaps not surprising, as its creation was strongly linked to the political currents of the time, but I think that care must be taken to introduce changes on the basis of new insights backed up by research evidence, or pragmatic experience, rather than on the basis of political ideology.

There are also philosophical differences between the British NHS and the Dutch Health Service, especially in relation to issues like euthanasia and drug addiction. However, there also appear to be remarkable similarities with regard to the philosophy of care in the community.

All things considered, the role of the psychologist in Britain is not much different to that of a psychologist in the Netherlands, although there are small differences in the various specialisms of the profession. We also have the help of psychological assistants (not the same thing as assistant psychologists over here) who have been thoroughly trained in psychometrics and whose job is specifically to do psychological testing.

All in all, moving to another country was a big step but I feel it was worth it. First, I am able to work as a psychologist, whereas many of my Dutch colleagues are still struggling to gain employment. Although it has been remarked that I would probably have a higher income in the

Netherlands (if a job were to be available) the cost of living and taxes are lower in Britain, so one cancels out the other nicely. Furthermore, living and working in another country is a worthwhile experience in itself, as it opens up new insights into life as well as work.'

Robin Paijmans, Psychologist, Hull and Holderness Community Health NHS Trust.

Free movement – the reality

As already stated, the mobility of workers across European borders is currently a trickle rather than a flood, despite the '1992' programme which aimed to dismantle internal barriers to free movement. There are many reasons for this, one major obstacle for British workers being the language barrier. Another is the simple lack of awareness and the lack of perception, so clearly stated by Robin Paijmans of the Netherlands, that Europe is an open market for job seekers. Many British job seekers, whether employed people seeking promotion or a change of career, or unemployed people simply seeking work, do not think of looking outside the UK (with the well known exception of the construction industry). Traditionally, those who do so have tended to settle in another English-speaking country, either as expatriates or as immigrants, if they can secure legal status. However, there has been a noticeable shift in recent years, with European Union countries becoming more popular destinations than former colonies, though there is currently no way of knowing if this trend will continue or even if those concerned will prove to be long-term migrants.

Mobile Britons seem to be choosing Germany as their favourite destination, with over 100 000 British-born people currently resident there. In comparison, only 42 000 Germans are living in the UK. The Irish Republic is second choice, but a long way behind at 58 000, and France comes third, with 50 000 Britons currently in residence. However, freedom of movement is likely to encourage short-term emigration simply because it is so much easier now to make the transition to an EU country, and consequently easy to move back again. This may change gradually as the insularity of certain nations (particularly the British) decreases. Those who are sufficiently adventurous to seek work in another country are at present acting as pioneers and through them, many of the barriers to mobility are being exposed and addressed. The mobile workers of the future will consequently find their paths smoothed.

This is particularly true of the difficulties surrounding the issue of transparency of qualifications, where obstacles have stubbornly remained in place despite the various actions taken at European level. Even those professionals covered by the 'sectoral' directives and with systems of recognition dating back to the 1970s are not moving freely. Bureaucracy and red tape in some countries is often simply too much for prospective job seekers and there have also been examples of blatant discrimination against nationals of other Member States, possibly due to protectionist policies. A Belgian nurse was refused permanent employment in France in 1986 on the grounds that nurses were civil servants and only French nationals could work in the civil service – hence the exclusion. The law found against France on this occasion, but a number of other objections have continued to be raised by French employing authorities against other applicants. In several Member States, bureaucratic delays caused by the insistence on applicants producing a variety of documents or undergoing tests at designated hospitals have also been widely experienced. Where a profession is unregulated in a Member State – for instance chiropody in Greece – the theory is that job applicants do not have to apply for mutual recognition of their qualifications and should be considered under the same conditions applying to host state nationals. In reality, the applicant may find him or herself in the same position as the starship *USS Enterprise*, having to 'boldly go' where no chiropodist has gone before.

Even those who emerge from this ordeal still intent on employment in their chosen country may find that they are ill-prepared for work there. Unfortunately, because so little comparable information exists, it is not always possible to prepare individuals for the differences in practices and procedures they may experience in a foreign country. Information provided on salaries in different countries can be quite misleading, with complicated formulae relating to age, qualifications, years of service, etc. affecting rates of pay. Working conditions can also be different to what is perceived as the norm by 'foreign' workers. This can lead to dissatisfaction and an inability to remain in post and fulfil contracts. For example, a German hospital which recruited 30 nurses in 1993 via a recruitment agency was disappointed to find that only two remained in post by the end of the year.

Some professional groups are making efforts to overcome this obstacle, for example, the occupational therapists, who have produced a code of ethics and standards for the profession and whose professional association disseminates European-wide data on OT training and practice. Useful work is also being done by bodies such as the Nursing and Midwifery unit at WHO's Regional Office for Europe, where staff have been compiling Nursing Profiles to help make the roles and responsibilities of nurses and midwives in Europe more transparent. Even where practices, procedures and role functions are similar and well understood, transferring skills from one country to another is not an instantaneous process. For one thing, those expecting to achieve their accustomed standards and outcomes in a culturally different environment are simply not being realistic; workers do not perform in a vacuum, and the standards and procedures of the host culture will inevitably become those of the newly-introduced worker. Workers who succeed in making the transition to another country also find that they need a period of adjustment during which they redevelop their professional competence to their accustomed levels of dexterity and speed, within the unfamiliar environment. Skills and professional competence are acquired within a specific context; when the context changes radically, there must be an acclimatization period. This is often difficult for many experienced professionals to accept.

More information about working conditions and practices in other countries would assist those thinking of moving to take up posts elsewhere in Europe, but this is scarce and what exists is not easily accessible to the working practitioner. Some health care professionals may even discover that their specialist profession is not actually recognized as such in the country to which they intend to move, or is not regarded as a specialist area in its own right. In the case of nursing, for example, few nurses outside the UK are specifically trained as specialists in psychiatry or in mental illness. In countries where these specialisms exist, they are frequently in the form of additional training and qualifications as opposed to the UK system of nurse preparation.

Within the medical profession, the term 'specialist' is itself the subject of debate. In the UK, the concept of specialist grades was unknown amongst doctors, who became consultants in their specialist fields in response to service needs, rather than as a gradual progression through a recognized process of specialization. As a result of the right to freedom of movement, doctors from other European community countries were asking to be recognized as specialists when seeking employment in the UK, and were finding their paths blocked by the existing system.

As a consequence of this, a Working Group was set up to investigate and make recommendations on specialist training and recognition in the UK. The *Report of the Working Group on Specialist Medical Training, 1993* (commonly known as the 'Calman Report') recommended that a Certificate in Specialist Training should be introduced. Holders of the certificate, and of similar appropriate certificates from other Member States, should be indicated on the Medical Register by the initials 'CT'. These recommendations are only now being implemented, following agreement with the Royal Colleges and professional organizations; therefore anomalies still exist, such as the treatment within the UK and Ireland of genitourinary medicine and dermatology as separate disciplines, which in other EU countries are a joint speciality, 'dermatovenereology'.

In the face of such problems, many professional groups believe that more guidance and information is needed at EU level and that the European Commission should actively facilitate free movement, rather than provide the framework for it to occur.

Despite all the barriers, there are clearly opportunities and benefits for those willing to accept the challenges. Although there are many instances of over supply of health care workers

– for example, doctors in Spain – in reality there are often frequent regional scarcities, linked to speciality. There are also very definite areas where countries are experiencing difficulty in supplying certain professional groups. Here in the UK, for example, we have a shortage of physiotherapists, whereas nurses with specialist skills in theatre and intensive care will have little difficulty in finding suitable employment in Germany and several other EU countries. Obviously, skills shortages vary from State to State and those wishing to take advantage of free movement would do well to monitor them before making any physical moves.

Some future implications of free movement of people

There are obvious social implications arising from more common and widespread mobility, such as increased isolation of family members and the effects of a more mobile population on communities. Some of the economic implications have also been mentioned, such as the potential opportunity to purchase services more cheaply, and the differences in salary levels between countries. The reaction of the nursing profession to the introduction of locally-negotiated pay in 1995 was an indication of how strongly a particular group felt about the need to maintain nationally-agreed levels of professional remuneration for their work. One of the reasons for this was that highly qualified nurses could gravitate towards services paying the most. The consequence could be that deprived areas with insufficient funds available to provide high salaries would be unable to attract high-calibre staff.

A European pay structure for health and welfare professionals is a long way off, and indeed, may never materialize. However, economic factors are one of the most powerful motives for geographical mobility and once professional mobility begins to take effect, workers will inevitably converge on employers offering the best salaries and conditions.

Information for the mobile worker: the European Employment Services Network (EURES)

EURES was established in 1993 to provide information about the EU labour market and to inform and advise individuals about living and working conditions in the Member States. It also disseminates information about job offers, via its network of Euroadvisers. There will ultimately be 400 of these, linked by a computer network and able to access a central database hosted by the European Commission's INFO 92 system. (A list of Euroadvisers in the UK can be found in the Resource section at the back of this book.)

However, the service offered by EURES is not well known, at least in the UK, and enquirers are usually referred by the Employment Service rather than approaching their local Euroadvisers direct. This is a pity, because not only does EURES provide services for the individual, it also produces useful documentation on individual European countries and general working conditions there. (In order to live and work in another country, it is obviously essential for workers to understand areas like education and taxation, as well as social security systems, and the range of benefits available. This is particularly true for health care professionals because they not only need to be able to participate as citizens of the host country themselves but to understand the attitudes, pressures and concerns of patients and service users.) The service is likely to develop a higher profile in the future and become more widely used.

Freedom of movement – who is responsible for making it happen?

Despite the efforts made to open up the European Union to its own citizenry, barriers to widespread free movement of people will take a long time to disappear. The culture of mobility has yet to become part of British consciousness as far as the general public is concerned. In fact, few European nations can be said to regard the EU as an open labour market, given the low numbers of workers taking advantage of freedom of movement. If this is to change, more effort must be made by the European Commission to provide the necessary information and assistance and to 'police' the system, and Member State governments must co-operate fully and cease protectionist and bureaucratic practices. However, the responsibility does not lie solely with the European institutions and national governments alone. People must not only be aware of the opportunities open to them and willing to embrace new cultures and new ways of life, they must be confident enough in their professional abilities and their transferable skills to know that they will be capable of doing so. The responsibility for ensuring that they gain these qualities must therefore be shared between policy makers and practitioners concerned with all forms of education, training and personal and professional development.

Summary points

1 Freedom of movement of people is multi-dimensional – freedom to live and work in another Member State of the Union is central, but movement as part of education and training, the movement of information and ideas, and medical tourism are also involved.

2 All citizens of the European Union have the right to move to another EU country and seek work there, but relatively few people are doing so at present. For the UK, the barriers of insularity, language, culture and limited perception are still marked.

3 Some people with certain qualifications will find their paths smoothed by legislation, EU efforts to create enabling frameworks and by agreements between professional bodies. Others will still have to persuade prospective employers of their professional competence themselves, taking account of the fact that occupational arrangements can vary quite considerably between Member States.

4 There are various things that people wishing to work elsewhere in the EU can do to take the initiative and help themselves, but good preparation is essential.

5 The situation should become easier and more straightforward as time goes on and employers become more familiar and comfortable with the idea of employing 'foreign' workers. There will also be new ways of achieving transparency between qualifications.

6 All health care workers, particularly those in public health and health care management, will in future need the skills and breadth of vision to operate on a broader canvas. This will include an awareness of major developments and conditions across Europe – how health, social and environmental services are organized and how they are affected by socio-cultural differences. So far the professional and regulatory bodies have continued to focus primarily on UK health issues, but the pre-service sector is taking a lead by Europeanizing the curriculum and encouraging students to undertake exchanges and study visits.

7 Most of the impetus for change in attitude and practice has come from the field, often emerging from the first hand experience of health care professionals.

8 Professional networking and collaboration on curriculum development and training has not been the norm to date, but is capable of bearing valuable fruit.

9 The complexity of European health workforce planning has been a neglected field. The broader human resource issues of skill mix, volume, cost and conditions may have been considered nationally, but there is little evidence of strategic thinking being done within the European context, even for something as fundamental as staff supply and demand. As a result, there is a lack of quality information easily available to staff on the ground.

10 The European Employment Services Network (EURES) deserves to be better known and utilized.

11 In the face of so many problems, breakthrough may be dependent upon the Union actively facilitating free movement, rather than just attempting to set up frameworks for it to occur.

References and further reading

Buchan, J., Seccombe, I. and Ball, J. (1992). *The International Mobility of Nurses: a UK Perspective*. Institute of Manpower Studies, Report No. 230.

Communication on recognition of qualifications for academic and professional purposes. COM (94) 596 final. Commission of the European Communities.

Creating Lifelong Learners: partnerships for care. (1994). Guidelines for midwifery and nursing. Programmes of education leading to registration. English National Board of Nursing, Midwifery and Health Visiting.

Key data on education in the European Union, 1995. (1994) Office for Official Publications of the European Communities.

The Health Sector in the European Community – 1992 and Beyond. (1991). Discussion paper from the European Foundation for the Improvement of Living and Working Conditions.

Ness, M., Cutter, J. and Johnson, S. (1993). *Towards a Single European Market: A Case Study of Nursing*. Yorkshire Regional Health Authority. (Copies available from: Sue Hamer, The Institute of Nursing, University of Leeds, 18 Blenheim Terrace, Leeds LS2 9HD. Fax 0113 2422411).

Pritchard, A.P. and Wallace, M.J. (1994). *Accident and Emergency Nursing*.

The Single Market – Europe Open for Professions. (1992). The Department of Trade and Industry and the central office of information.

Versieck, K., Bouten, R. and Pacolet, J. (1995). *Manpower Problems in the Nursing/Midwifery Professions in the EC*. The Hospital Committee of the European Community.

Williams, Sir David Innes (1992). *Healthcare Delivery in the European Community Conference proceedings, Standards of Excellence* series. NHS Training Directorate, Bristol.

Appendix 1: Personal checklist for health care workers considering professional mobility

- Start preparation early;
- Consider your current language competence and prepare accordingly;
- Set up some work experience or a study visit well in advance of any move;
- Collect all information available about your destination and occupation by contacting/visiting:
    libraries and book shops
    the appropriate embassy

relevant professional bodies both in the UK and your
chosen country (e.g. RCN)
tourist information offices
professional journals and publications
the EURES Euroadviser service (which produces *Working In* ... booklets).

- Undertake some focused reading on the health care system
  of your chosen country, policies and practices, salaries and
  conditions, etc. If possible contact regional or national
  bodies concerned with labour market intelligence to identify
  if there is an under or over supply in your specialism;
- Check out your position with regard to the mutual
  recognition of qualifications by contacting your regulatory
  body (if appropriate);
- Request information from the Department of Social
  Security and the Inland Revenue;
- Consult the NATVACs lists (National Vacancies), which
  should be available in job centres;
- Find and speak to a member of your profession with
  experience of working in your country of destination, or,
  failing that, a member of another health care profession;
- Arrange a cultural briefing, preferably from someone native
  to your country of destination but living in the UK;
- Make a list of all the other things you need to check, such as
  if you need a work permit or residence permit, professional
  liability insurance as well as personal insurance, licensing of
  your car (if you are taking it with you), etc.;
- Speak to your Euroadviser again about specific issues once
  you are fully briefed.

Appendix 2: The Council's standards for education experience outside the UK for students undertaking national board approved programmes leading to registration or recording on the Council's register

Principles of provision of experience outside the UK

1 The provision of experience outside the UK must be based on the following principles:

1.1 the experience outside the UK must be congruent with the overall programme leading to registration, or recording in the UK;

1.2 individualized learning outcomes must be agreed for the period of experience;

1.3 appropriate preparation of the student must be made to ensure that the maximum gain is achieved from the experience;

1.4 personal support must be provided to facilitate the student experience;

1.5 a named supervisor/mentor from the host country must be attached to the student for the duration of the experience and

1.6 a clear delineation between observational and direct care experience must be made.

Nature of experience

2 The nature of experience could be either observational or direct care, or combinations of the two may occur. Programme planners must be clear about the objectives of the experience and plan the content accordingly. All programmes must be based on the principles set out in paragraph 1 above.

Learning outcomes

Observational only placements

3 The experience should offer the student the opportunity to:

3.1 gain an understanding of the philosophy and value of systems underpinning nursing, midwifery and/or health visiting in another country;

3.2 acquire an understanding of the points of similarity and contrast between nursing, midwifery and/or health visiting in two or more countries; and

3.3 critically examine and evaluate comparative methods of delivery of care.

Direct care placements

4 In addition to the outcomes set out in 3, the experience should offer the student the opportunity to:

4.1 gain experience not readily available in the UK; and/or

4.2 gain a wider perspective of health care and its delivery outside the UK; and

4.3 participate in the delivery of nursing, midwifery and/or health visiting care outside the UK.

Length of experience

5 Observation only placements should not normally exceed two weeks in length.

6 Direct care placements should not normally exceed 10 per cent of the total programme approved by a National Board for registration or recording in the UK.

Reproduced with the kind permission of the United Kingdom Central Council for Nursing, Midwifery and Health Visiting.

8

European-funded programmes – a pot of gold in Brussels?

Aims of this Chapter

In this chapter, we aim to:
- challenge some of the myths about European funding;
- explain where it comes from;
- outline the rationale and aims behind European funding and its relationship with policies;
- briefly describe some specific programmes;
- give examples of how the money has been used.

European funding – getting it into perspective

This book is not an instruction manual on how to secure funding from European institutions, though such documents do exist and can be useful if viewed within the right context. This is essentially that European policies are more important than funded programmes, which are merely the mechanisms by which policies are implemented. Unfortunately, this is not the view of many organizations and individuals (especially consultants), who are so keen to get their hands on the 'pot of gold' in Brussels that they fail to recognize the policy issues which are the *raison d'être* for the funding in the first place.

This is a problem, because such a perception means that

policy issues are not being properly discussed or considered by organizations, simply because they regard European activities as being primarily grant-related. Many of the posts associated with European work in the public sector are funding-related, and the job descriptions applying to them are peppered with references to identifying sources of funding that can be exploited, making applications or bids for funding, or working on income-generational initiatives. Policy matters are often relegated to the bottom of the list or mentioned as an afterthought – if at all.

Additionally, most organizations – especially those cash-starved public or voluntary sector bodies which are becoming increasingly desperate for funding to stay afloat – want money to do the things that are *their* priorities, not those which are necessarily the priorities of the European Union institutions. For European projects, the best possible scenario is a close match between the two sets of priorities, culminating in a useful activity which results in real benefit for the communities involved and is transferable across the EU. The worst scenario is that a project is established simply to attract funding, money may even be claimed for activities which have not occurred, and the cash simply feeds into an organization's beleaguered budget. These are the two extremes; the reality is usually somewhere in the middle.

Securing funding from 'Europe' is also by no means an easy option. For one thing, most of the monies disbursed via EU programmes is in the form of matched funding, rather than a 100 per cent grant with no strings attached. Programme criteria require the organization involved to make a financial or resource commitment itself to the project. In addition, there are detailed criteria for eligibility and often a considerable extra administrative burden. Many programmes require a 'transnational' focus or at the very least a transnational element, and this, too, is becoming more rigorously defined and scrutinized.

However, once they recognize the issues involved, organizations should not be deterred from securing funding from European Union sources. In fact, European projects and the transnational partnerships they usually require can result in a significant enhancement of an organization's activities, be of real value to the staff or students participating and be very enjoyable experiences in their own right. To achieve this, European transnational project work should be seen specifically as an enhancement to existing activities, and as an additional enabling element. A project itself should never be undertaken solely for the sake of the funding it brings, nor should the organization's activities be funding-driven. At the very least, to undertake a project simply to bring in money can have the effect of dissipating the resources and energies of the organization, and at worst, distorting its core activity.

It is important to stress the need to influence future policy and help shape future funding programmes. Health care organizations should be not simply trying to fit into existing European funding programmes but actively influencing the European Commission and others to ensure that adequate funding is made available to address EU competence in the field of health provision . Unless the European Commission is made aware of the interests of health care organizations throughout Europe, it will not be in a position to ensure that European strategies are effective and relevant (this will be discussed in more detail in Chapter 9).

Although European funded programmes may appear superficially to be numerous and diverse, they are in fact all contributory parts of strategic plans for achieving policy aims. Within each family or group of programmes during a particular timescale, the intention is to address certain identified priority areas, and the Commission is a great believer in synergy (i.e. the idea that the combined effects of a number of programmes or actions, properly co-ordinated, can exceed the impact of a plethora of individual, unco-ordinated actions). For instance, the creation of an 'information society' is an objective which is either central or peripheral to several funded programmes, and of generic benefit to many sectors within industry or the public sector. In this way, the intention is that European policy issues are implemented via a number of ways and in various contexts, which combine to have a fundamental impact on society and the economy as a whole.

European funding – where does it come from?

Far from being fairy gold at the end of the rainbow, the budget of the European Union is financed by various means, all of them boringly prosaic. One major source is via a share of VAT collected from Member States, and another is customs duties and agricultural levies on imported (i.e. from outside the EU) products. In addition, each Member State also contributes a share based on its Gross National Product (GNP), but this accounts for only 20.9 per cent of the EU budget. Amounts are highly variable: in 1994, the UK contribution amounted to 11.6 per cent of the EU general budget, whilst Italy contributed 14.1 per cent and France 19.2 per cent. Germany's contribution represented 30.1 per cent of the budget.

The EC budget has long been the subject of controversy. The budget itself is drafted by the European Commission, but it must be agreed by the Parliament and then by the Council of Ministers before it can be finalized. Each of the latter institutions has its own agenda, the Parliament's usually being to boost the budget and emphasize European unity, increasing activities and initiatives, whilst the Council of Ministers often tends towards minimizing expenditure at EU level, perceiving issues more from a national government view.

Something which has long been a major cause for concern has been the high level of support for agriculture, coupled with the over-production which has occurred for a number of years. We are all familiar with the newspaper horror stories associated with the Common Agricultural Policy (CAP), dealing with wine lakes and cauliflower mountains, which have helped to discredit the competence of the European institutions in the eyes of the British public. The ongoing reform of the CAP attempts to tackle this, but agriculture still accounts for a significant share of the EU budget (49.3 per cent in 1994). However, as the Commission points out, Member States would need to support their agricultural sectors themselves if the CAP did not exist and other major economies like Japan and the US have similar programmes of support for their farmers. Nevertheless, the CAP continues to be a source of controversy whenever the EU budget is discussed, and has been frequently cited by Eurosceptics as a major financial burden on UK taxpayers.

Another popular misconception is that a large part of the EU budget is swallowed up by the Brussels bureaucracy. In fact, administration accounts for only 4.8 per cent, despite the requirement for considerable numbers of interpreters and translation facilities.

The 'structural funds'

After the funding allocated to farm subsidies and the like under the Common Agricultural Policy, the largest items on the EU budget are the Structural Funds. The Funds are so called because they are intended to tackle disparities in wealth and economic prosperity by improving both the infrastructure and education and training provision in areas which are underdeveloped or in need of assistance because they are disadvantaged in some way (e.g. as a result of the decline of traditional industries such as coal and steel, or fisheries). The idea is that structural change can be effected by ensuring that the lower-achieving economies of the EU are brought nearer to the level of the high achievers, so that the European Union as a whole will ultimately become a cohesive and highly developed economic global power.

One of the Funds relates to agriculture (the European Agricultural Guidance and Guarantee Fund) and is unlikely to be of interest to health care professionals. The other two Funds are the European Regional Development Fund (ERDF) and the European Social Fund (ESF). The Funds underwent a fundamental reform in 1988, and were reviewed again prior to the current phase of 1994–99, when only minor changes were made. The Regulations governing the Funds were adopted on 20 July 1993, when the Funds were granted a budget of 141 billion ECU.

Eligibility for assistance under the Structural Funds is related to specific objectives defined at European level. They are:

• Objective 1: improving the development of regions which are under-developed;

- Objective 2: regenerating designated areas affected by industrial decline;
- Objective 3: combating long-term unemployment and assisting young people into work; helping those exposed to exclusion from the labour market; and promoting equal opportunities between men and women;
- Objective 4: providing support for workers having to adapt to industrial change;
- Objective 5(b): promoting the development of rural areas.

Criteria set out for the objectives define those regions within the EU which are eligible, where the criteria relate to certain geographical conditions. Those which qualify for 'Objective 1' status usually benefit most from EU funding.

One of the fundamental principles of the revised structural funds, and indeed of most European financial assistance, is that the monies allocated should be additional to those already provided by national, regional or local governments. In other words, European funds should not be used instead of government funding, or to make savings for governments in their own budgets. (This has been the source of some difficulties between the UK government and the European Commission in the past.) The concept of 'additionality' was especially defined in 1988, to clarify this position.

According to the Regulation, 'In order to achieve a genuine economic impact, the Structural Funds ... may not replace public expenditure on structural or comparable expenditure undertaken by the Member State in the whole of the territory eligible under an objective. For this purpose ... the Commission and the Member State concerned shall ensure that the Member State maintains, in the whole of the territory concerned, its public structural or comparable expenditure at least at the same level as in the previous programming period.' (Council Regulation (EEC) No. 2082/93, 20 July 1993, Article 9. Official Journal No. 193, 31-7-93.)

In other words, the Structural Funds should not be used as replacements for 'core' public spending by Member State governments and the resultant savings used to finance their own policy priorities, or tax cuts, for example. The additionality principle was tightened up when the Structural

Funds were reformed in 1988 because of the problems the
Commission had previously encountered in making Member
States adhere to it. They must now provide evidence to verify
additionality at the stage when they submit their plans and
again during implementation.

ERDF funding is mainly used to match public sector
funding for capital costs of projects relating to the infrastructure, whilst ESF grant aid provides revenue funding for
activities such as training courses. Unlike most other EU-
funded programmes, there is no requirement for projects
funded under the structural funds to be 'transnational'.

'Community initiatives'

A range of other programmes are funded out of the same
budgets as the Structural Funds but are separate from them in
the sense that they are initiatives specially designated at
European level and benefiting a particular group or addressing
a specific problem. The 'Community initiatives' are intended
to facilitate innovative developments, often transnational
projects which enable organizations across the EU to work
together, to find transferable solutions to common concerns.
Several are linked to regional aid, and these may only be open
to eligible regions or countries. Others target declining
industries needing to diversify and revitalize their economies.
Yet another group are the 'human resource' initiatives and
these are the most likely to be of interest to health care
professionals.

Employment Horizon is a programme concerned with
assisting the integration into the labour market of people
excluded by disadvantages of various kinds, including
disabilities.

Employment Now is aimed specifically at women and is
intended to reduce unemployment and assist women to
become economically active in various ways, often via training
schemes or guidance facilities.

Employment Youthstart targets young people, especially
under the age of 20, and aims to provide access to employment
or recognized forms of education and training.

In addition, there is a Community initiative called **Adapt**, which aims to help workers adapt to industrial and technological change. All of these initiatives are administered by the Department for Education and Employment (see the Resource section for contacts).

Activities funded are extremely varied, but all proposed projects must receive public authority support in the form of matched funding in order to be eligible for European funding.

Transnationality

Certain programmes require that activities funded under them must be 'transnational': in other words, projects must be jointly carried out by partnerships involving organizations from several Member States, working together. The idea is to spread best practice, exchange ideas and develop an understanding of the different approaches and attitudes involved. Unfortunately, a number of these partnerships have in the past been established simply to comply with funding criteria, and no real collaborative work has been undertaken.

Education and training: the foundation stone of the Union?

The importance of education and training in building Europe's economic and social prosperity has been emphasized repeatedly by the European institutions. It is a principle which is firmly embedded in the national consciousness of certain European countries, and the northern Member States generally have had higher participation rates in further and higher education than the UK. In fact, only Portugal has a lower participation rate in higher education than the UK, with 9 per cent of the population involved in higher education in 1991/2 compared with the UK's 11 per cent, the same as Greece. Italy, Denmark and Germany all had rates of 16 per cent. (Luxembourg's 2 per cent is misleading because most of its students go abroad to study.) (*Key data on education in the European Union, 1994*, 1995.)

A commitment to investment in education and training at all levels is being actively encouraged by the EU, supported by funded programmes linked to specific policy areas and identified priorities. One of these is the 'European dimension' in education and training programmes. This 'European dimension' has been recognized by a wide range of UK-based organizations, such as the (former) Department for Education, which issued guidance to schools on integrating a European dimension into schools and colleges. The Open University has a modular course entitled *Learning Through Life: Education and Training Beyond School* which places the adult learner within a European context and includes a European File, with information and views from European practitioners and learners. Some organizations are now incorporating a European dimension in their own staff development and in-service training programmes.

What is a European dimension?

Integrating a European dimension can be as simple as perceiving the individual or organization within a wider European context, rather than a purely national one. This approach is a natural state of mind in many European countries, and seeing things within a European context is taken for granted. In the UK, we are not noted for developing a personal or organizational European consciousness – in other words, we don't feel ourselves to be European. We often talk about 'Europe' when we mean the continent of Europe, separate from the UK, clearly not feeling Britain to be part of Europe as we speak. Even within some large organizations, particularly in the public sector, strategic planning is undertaken from a purely insular perspective, rather than taking account of the wider European Union context.

In the UK, the European dimension has perhaps been most strongly emphasized in the private sector, partly due to the Single Market awareness-raising programmes led by the Department of Trade and Industry (DTI). This tended to focus on export-related issues, but also placed heavy emphasis on the need for skills development, particularly in languages.

(The point being that you cannot sell to people in anything but their own language – the monolingual sales representative has a limited career in a Europe without frontiers.)

In the field of education, the impetus for a European dimension came initially from the European institutions, and the high-profile treatment funded by the DTI was not matched by a similar awareness-raising campaign by the Department for Education. In 1988, the EC Council and the Ministers of Education meeting within the Council adopted a Resolution on the European dimension in Education. The purposes of the Resolution included the strengthening of a sense of European identity for students, as well as improving their knowledge of the EC, etc. Member States were required to formulate policies on incorporating the European dimension in education and the UK government published a policy statement in 1991, which again stressed the need for development of a sense of European identity. (This concern with creating and embedding a sense of European identity bore fruit within the Maastricht Treaty, which established rights for European citizens which are additional to their rights as citizens of their own Member States.)

In 1992, the then Department of Education and Science (DES) issued a guidance document on the European dimension. Its full title was *Policy Models: A Guide to Developing and Implementing European Dimension Policies in LEAs, Schools and Colleges*. The 'key factors for success' listed within it included 'a co-ordinated programme of professional development'. Also mentioned was the need for specific skills such as competence in other European languages.

As indicated in Chapter 6, staff responsible for development and training for those preparing to work in the field of health and social care are now beginning to incorporate a European dimension to their curricula, and linking this with opportunities for work experience or periods of study abroad, often funded under EU programmes. They are also looking to provide in-service training and professional updating for professionals.

The education and training of health professionals is one of the issues considered in the European Commission's *Communication on the framework for action in the field of public health*

(COM(3)559) published by the Commission of the European Communities. The Communication recognizes the vital role health care professionals can play in helping to shape a future European health policy and specific reference is made in the Communication to their education and training needs. For its part, the Commission will 'try to increase the effectiveness of the health professional's role in public health, evaluate existing courses, collaborate on new ones promoted and foster exchanges of experiences and information on teaching and training'.

European programmes for education and training

European education and training activities and initiatives have undergone a thorough evaluation and have now been reorganized into two main programmes in line with Articles 126 and 127 of the Treaty of European Union. Article 126 states that 'The Community shall contribute to the development of quality education by encouraging co-operation between Member States, and, if necessary, by supporting and supplementing their action ...' whilst Article 127 states that 'The Community shall implement a vocational training policy which shall support and supplement the action of the Member States...'.

The two programmes are **Socrates**, which covers educational activities, and **Leonardo da Vinci**, which incorporates several types of activity relating to vocational training.

Socrates

The European education initiatives are made up of a combination of different strands within the overall Socrates programme. There are three main spheres of action within the programme: higher education, school education and 'horizontal actions' relating to language teaching, open and distance learning and exchanges of information and advice.

Some activities already existed and have been simply modified or adapted, whilst others are completely new areas. (One of the latter is the school-related stand of the programme, which has been given the name Comenius.) Most of the budget for Socrates is concentrated on the higher education activities. The programme will be reviewed after three years of operation.

As with many other programmes, the activities funded under Socrates are transnational and projects involve several European countries working co-operatively to achieve identified aims which are in line with the programme's goals.

Leonardo da Vinci

Training programmes have been similarly grouped together under the programme known as Leonardo da Vinci. The overall goal of the programme is to improve the quality of vocational training systems and their innovative capacity, in order to produce a workforce ready for the technological challenges of the twenty-first century. It takes forward some of the programmes which existed previously and builds on them further, and also introduces new elements.

One of the central themes of the Leonardo programme is 'lifelong learning', the idea that individuals need to develop an attitude towards training as something which is ongoing and continuous throughout their lives, rather than an activity which is of short duration and related to a particular phase (1996 has also been designated European Year of Lifelong Learning).

Previous schemes

A number of separate programmes existed prior to Socrates and Leonardo, most of which have been incorporated into the new programmes. They provided financial assistance for developmental work and for mobility of students and staff in educational institutions, as well as for 'young workers'. Health care professionals are amongst those who have benefited from these schemes in the past, and will continue to benefit in the future under Socrates, Leonardo and other EU programmes. The 'old' programmes – still familiar to many people – included:

- **Erasmus** (European Community Action Scheme for the Mobility of University Students). Launched in 1987, Erasmus enabled the establishment of Inter-university Co-operation Programmes (now numbering over 2500) and provided funding for students to study abroad, receiving academic recognition from the students' home university (it is now part of Socrates).
- **Comett** (University–Industry Co-operation in Technology Training). Launched in 1986, this was conceived as a training-oriented counterpart to the EC's Research and Development programmes, and aimed to expand co-operation between universities and industry and to improve the quality of technological training at a European level. Under this programme, organizations known as University–Enterprise Training Partnerships (UETPs) were set up across the EC, some general, some specializing in particular areas (now incorporated into Leonardo).
- **Eurotecnet** (Promotion of Innovation in Vocational Training related to Technological Change). Eurotecnet had a three-year preparatory phase before being formalized in 1990 as a support programme addressing the impact of technological change on qualification systems and on training methodologies (again, incorporated into Leonardo).
- **Force** (Action Programme for the Development of Continuing Vocational Training – based on a French acronym, *For*mation *C*ontinue en *E*urope). Force was established in 1991 and dealt with aspects of policy development, innovation and exchanges of experience and expertise in relation to continuing education and training (these will now be taken forward within the framework of the Leonardo programme).
- **Lingua** (Action Programme to Promote Foreign Language Competence in the EC). Launched in 1990, the Lingua programme focused on the need for more EC citizens to be able to communicate in an EC language other than their own, and provided for various training actions including the development of language materials and curricula and student and staff mobility (now part of Socrates).
- **Petra** (Vocational Training of Young People and Preparation for Working Life). This scheme, in existence

since 1988, developed from an earlier EC programme to assist the transition of young people from school to adult and working life. It was intended to take account in particular of problems related to high youth unemployment by setting EC standards for initial vocational training (initiatives developed under Petra are now part of Leonardo).

- **Tempus** (Trans-European Mobility Programme for University Students). Tempus was set up in 1990, to assist in the transformation of higher education systems in Central and Eastern European countries by means of co-operation in the development of new structures, systems and curricula, and through staff and student mobility. Note: Tempus forms part of the EC's overall provision of assistance to Central and Eastern Europe in the framework of the **Phare** programme – originally based on the acronym: *P*oland and *H*ungary – *A*ssistance for *R*egeneration of the *E*conomy – and similar arrangements have been established with the Republics of the Independent States via the **Tacis** programme (Technical Assistance to the CIS). Tempus (Tacis) extends to parts of the former Soviet Union: Russia, Ukraine and Belarus (from 1994) and Kazahkstan, Kyrghystan, Moldova and Uzbekistan (from 1995).

Most of these programmes came to the end of their funding cycle at the end of 1994 or early in 1995, and were replaced or integrated within the new Socrates and Leonardo pro-grammes, which are now well underway.

Equal opportunities for men and women

Within a European context, 'equal opportunities' refers to equality between men and women rather than the broad interpretation it has developed here in the UK, where it is perceived within the context of equal opportunities for ethnic minorities and disabled people as well as sex equality. The EU Equal Opportunities Action Programme, now scheduled to begin its fourth cycle (from 1996–2000), is aiming to emphasize the concept of 'mainstreaming' – that is, ensuring that equality of opportunity is integrated into all policy areas.

Programmes for people with disabilities and disadvantaged groups are separate and tend to be linked with other initiatives – for instance, the TIDE programme is part of the telematics RTD programme (outlined in the next section) and Employment Horizon is one of the Community initiatives, already described.

Research and development programmes

Another area of transnational co-operation encouraged and nurtured by the European Commission is research and technological development (RTD). The Commission believes that research and development is a key factor contributing to economic success, and the European Framework Programmes established for RTD are intended to maintain and strengthen the international competitiveness of European industry in high-tech sectors in the global marketplace, as well as improving the quality of life for EU citizens.

The Fourth Framework Programme (FP4) was agreed by the Council of Ministers on 26 April 1994. Again, the principle of subsidiarity is important for RTD and projects funded under this family of programmes should be of a kind which benefit from international co-operation. All projects have to demonstrate that they have a useful, transferable outcome or product, and that this product would eventually be viable in commercial production (if appropriate).

The individual programmes within the Fourth Framework are grouped around the following themes:

- information and communication technologies;
- industrial technologies;
- environment;
- life sciences and technologies;
- energy;
- transport;
- targeted socio-economic research.

Several of the programmes within these themes are of interest to the health care sector, the most obvious being the biotechnology and biomedicine and health programmes within the Life Sciences theme area. In addition, there are programmes grouped within other main themes such as those concerned with telematics for health and nuclear fission safety and safeguards.

The Biotechnology programme (**Biotech II**) has clearly identified priority areas, which are:

- cell factories;
- genome analysis;
- plant and animal biotechnology;
- cell communication in neurosciences;
- immunology and vaccinology;
- structural biology;
- pre-normative research, biodiversity and social acceptance;
- infrastructures.

Biomed II is the biomedicine and health programme and again concentrates on a number of identified priorities:

- research on AIDS, TB and other infectious diseases;
- cancer research;
- pharmaceutical research;
- brain research;
- human genome research;
- occupational and environmental health research;
- diseases which have a major socio-economic impact (cancer, AIDS, cardiovascular diseases, chronic diseases, ageing and related problems, and rare diseases);
- public health research;
- biomedical technology and engineering research;
- biomedical ethics research.

The **Telematics for Health** programme concentrates on the development of telematics (a combination of telecommunications and information technology) in the context of health, for example, linking doctors with patients in remote areas, networking of health professionals, on-line organ donor registries, etc. There is also a telematics programme to support the integration of disabled and elderly people (the **TIDE** programme) which is another strand within the larger telematics research and development programme.

Programmes are intended to be supportive of the same broad aims and applicants must be aware of the links between them, and between other European programmes. The various individual programmes do not start and finish at the same time but are spread out, with each one being the subject of a 'Call for Proposals' issued in the *Official Journal*. This can often allow little time to get an application in and most applicant organizations (usually universities) know beforehand that a Call is due, via their own networks and electronic mail. The Commission provides an on-line service, Cordis, which provides information about RTD programmes and related issues. (There is also a Cordis newsletter.)

Projects must be able to demonstrate, in their initial applications, that there is a genuine and demonstrable need or problem to be addressed, that the socio-economic impact of the development has been considered, that work will be based on transnational co-operation, with each partner organization's credentials being described and their contribution to the project outlined, and that careful thought has been given to eventual commercial exploitation.

Other health-related programmes

The policies described earlier, specifically in Chapters 5 and 6, are being implemented via programmes which either concentrate solely on one issue or priority area or adopt a more broad spectrum approach to a theme. As already explained, the EU has a role to play in promoting health protection but has also identified specific health 'scourges' which are the focus of particular attention. The health programmes reflect this dual approach.

Health promotion programme

A five-year programme of Community action on health promotion, information and training within the framework for action in the field of public health is due to start in 1996 and run until the year 2000. A budget of 35 million ECU has been set aside to support a variety of activities which aim to result in a high level of health protection. Activities should encourage:

- formation of health promotion policies and strategies in Member States, which support co-operative actions such as exchange of experience, pilot projects and networking;
- adoption of healthy lifestyles and behaviour patterns;
- increased awareness of health risk factors and ways of enhancing health;
- multi-disciplinary and inter-sectoral approaches to health promotion which take account of socio-economic factors and the environment, especially for disadvantaged groups.

Europe Against Cancer

The *Europe Against Cancer* programme will continue for another five years, with a total budget of 64 million ECU. The activities eligible for funding support include studies, pilot projects and reports and others which:

- help to prevent premature deaths and reduce cancer-related mortality and morbidity;
- promote the quality of life by improving general health and well-being of the population and particularly by minimizing the social and economic consequences of cancer;
- assist in the collection of data and information in particular to establish common objectives and standardize data;
- enable dissemination of effective practice and exchange of experience, including exchanges of health personnel;
- create information networks.

AIDS and other communicable diseases

The identification of AIDS as a major health scourge has resulted in specific action against the disease, but when the new programme was planned, it was also extended to other communicable diseases. Actions in relation to AIDS and HIV are concentrated on data collection, activities relating to children and young people, measures to prevent transmission, social and psychological assistance and the combating of discrimination. For the identified communicable diseases, measures will be linked to vaccination, network creation and development, information provision, education and training and early detection. Budget value: 49.6 million ECU.

European programme to combat drug dependence

A five-year programme to combat drug dependence has been proposed, with a budget of over 28 million ECU. The programme's aims are:

- to improve public awareness;
- to interface with other programmes to have maximum effect (synergy);
- to support activities focusing on young people (especially school age) and the dissemination of good practice with this age group.

Some examples of European programmes in action

The following accounts have been provided by professionals personally involved in the funded activities concerned. Each is an example of a different kind of funded activity or project but each illustrates the value and importance of a pan-European approach.

Example 1

The 'Telegastro' Project

Professor Tim de Dombal, of the Clinical Information Science Unit at the University of Leeds, writes about the 'Telegastro' Project, an example of an EU-funded project for informatics in medicine:

'The objectives of the Telegastro Project were threefold: to develop a "consensus view" for a specific area of health care – gastroenterology – in order to identify and measure good treatment in a widely agreed, standardised and reproducible form; to develop a Telematics product to disseminate this information; and to assess the reaction of users. The overall aim was to assist the spread of good practice so as to improve the level of clinical care on a wide scale, to the benefit of physician, patient and the public purse.

The problem for most doctors is that medical knowledge has increased greatly, but courses of training simply cannot include all the information now available, and their memories could not cope if they did. Using a telematics application – a suite of computer programs which can be easily accessed and updated – ensures that an enormous amount of information is available to health care professionals, very rapidly and in a user-friendly form. This not only assists the practitioner to make a diagnosis, but ensures that internationally-agreed standards, criteria and terminology are used, whilst at the same time allowing the inclusion of local expertise via a special 'local variants' facility.

Between 1992 and 1994, the Project met the challenge of creating an international consensus of opinion by involving virtually all the relevant European associations and utilising an independent International Evaluation Panel. A pan-European approach was justified by the fact that 45% of the population in EC countries is estimated to experience one or more gastroenterological symptoms each year, at an annual treatment cost of 10 billion ECU, and with 70 000–100 000 lives being lost annually to gastroenterological disease.

A careful methodology was necessary to contain and reflect the views of senior clinicians in the field of gastroenterology, given that consensus agreement was vital to the acceptance of the end product.

The resulting Telematics product was initially tested with over 150 end-user institutions in 42 countries, and is now ready for demonstration and exploitation. The power of this application is reflected in the success of trials to test the ability of new users to secure specific clinical information from the product, and the ability of non-medically qualified persons (mainly medical students) to manage a clinical situation with the aid of the product.

The prototype has been embedded in both hospital and university networks, and also accessed remotely via Ethernet; successfully demonstrating both a multi-user and a remote user capability.

At this comparatively early stage, the potential impact of the project can already be clearly discerned. For example, where young doctors have followed an agreed, peer-recommended *modus operandi* in relation to acute abdominal pain, diagnostic accuracy has improved by 20%, with an improvement in appropriate and timely appendicectomy rates from 45% to 70%, in hospitals throughout the EC. Use of a "Telegastro style" educational package has produced similar results in 12 000 patients across three hospitals. The use of a similar package has been shown to improve comparisons between centres and different countries, despite language barriers.

So far the Project has produced an important "leading edge" demonstrator and a template that can be applied to other clinical areas – providing a niche for European health care telematics. By 1999 it is expected to cover most, if not all, routine gastroenterological practice, to have penetrated the majority of Europe's hospitals, in various European languages and in a variety of formats, from simple MS-DOS to multimedia, and to have had tangible impact on the delivery, and evaluation, of health care in Europe.'

Professor Tim de Dombal, Clinical Information Science Unit, University of Leeds

Example 2

A British occupational therapist on Crete

Deborah Taylor, who works for Wakefield and Pontefract Community Health Trust, writes about her Petra-funded work experience project on the island of Crete:

'A European Action Group consisting of a Leeds Further Education College, and its partner organisations in Greece and Denmark set up a series of European placements for health professionals, drawing upon funding from the EC's Petra programme. Additional support was provided by the Yorkshire Regional Health Authority, and young professionals (28 or below) were invited to apply for eight-week placements.

My employers endorsed my application and granted me study leave. I completed my placement during October and November of 1994, on the Greek island of Crete, together with three nursing clinician colleagues. I was the first UK occupational therapist to be placed in Greece via the programme, and my experience consisted of a full-time work placement with additional language support and cultural briefings. I was given twenty hours of intensive tuition in Modern Greek and self-help learning materials were available during the four weeks prior to my visit.

I knew that Greece is a member of the World Federation of Occupational Therapists and later found that OTs had been trained there since 1978. However, I discovered that they were scarce creatures. Therapy and rehabilitation are relatively new concepts in rural Greece and the extended family retains a prominent caring role. In addition, I also experienced problems with the planning and monitoring of the programme and the co-ordination between the UK placement organisers and their Greek contacts. My professional training, interests and experience were outlined in my application and in material taken to Crete, but where no direct equivalent existed, the information was not used to identify an alternative which was really suitable. The UK contacts relied upon individual contacts in Greece and there was a lack of comprehensive knowledge of the island's range of services. My colleagues and I were viewed with disapproval when we suggested transferring to different services, away from the host hospital designated. We were not expected to take responsibility for our own learning, and there were sometimes misunderstandings and conflict when we tried to negotiate alternative placements of more immediate relevance or offering a wider perspective.

When placed on an overcrowded general medical ward, assisting with designated practical tasks, I felt deskilled and disempowered. At times I was restricted by communication difficulties and misunderstanding of my role, and there was a strong ethic of attending work for a set number of hours despite the inertia I felt. However, people were determined to overcome these barriers, and the invitations we received to participate in the cultural life of our hosts were unconditional and warm. Ten days spent on Accident and Emergency also offered a real slice of life and an overview of the acute problems suffered.

Practical support was given to facilitate our visits to other services across the island. The British clinical adviser visited us in the penultimate week and was able to network on our behalf, securing a week's placement for me with Danaë, the OT at the University Hospital, who happened to be English-speaking. Danaë had established the service for in-patient care for 500 beds and initial input to Mental Health Services. She was also involved in developing educational software packages and is part of a European Database Project involving therapists from twelve countries. She told me that there were seven OTs in the city, with further developments with psychological services. It appeared that treatment and rehabilitation in physical medicine was far more sophisticated and socially acceptable than that related to the areas of mental health or learning disabilities.

By the end of my placement I had visited five centres outside our main city bases, including residential and treatment centres for children, a mental health institution and a primary health care clinic. I met some extremely well-motivated therapists who sought to update and improve their knowledge. The Greek Association (of occupational therapists) held their seminar in Athens the weekend I left (all such courses were self-financed).

The frustrations I have expressed did not detract from the value of the opportunity, nor the fond memories I retain about the experience. I had to adapt to a different culture – in fact, a different alphabet – and though the opportunity to speak English obviously led to more efficient communication, many other conversations I had were also rich and memorable.

I believe that worker mobility is important and that more employers should support it, utilising schemes like this, but always ensuring there is sufficient preliminary research and clear definition of working or study areas. The benefits include personal development, improved observation and evaluation skills, application to issues of ethnic minority groups accessing UK-based healthcare, building networks and exchanging ideas.'

Deborah Taylor, Senior Occupational Therapist, Regional Forensic Services (Mental Health), Wakefield and Pontefract Community Health NHS Trust

Example 3

Europe Against Cancer – **the Eccles Breast Cancer Screening Programme**

Professor J.T. Ennis, of the Institute of Radiological Sciences in Dublin, writes about his experience of the *Europe Against Cancer* programme:

'The Eccles Breast Screening Programme began as a Pilot Study in breast cancer screening, to establish the feasibility of ultimately introducing a more comprehensive, and eventually national, screening programme into Ireland. At that time, mammography was infrequently used in Ireland as a diagnostic method for detecting breast cancer. There was little expertise in either Radiology or Radiography, and there was little emphasis on quality assurance in relation to mammography technology.

The Pilot Study was part of a European initiative to reduce mortality from breast cancer. The aim was to establish pilot screening studies in those European countries where they did not currently exist. The countries that were selected included France, Belgium, Spain, Portugal, Greece and Ireland. While mammography was widely practised in some of these countries (i.e. France, Belgium and Spain), screening mammography had not been introduced as a specific technique for reducing mortality. Later, Italy joined the initiative, with the Screening Programme in Florence becoming part of the pilot network, which operated under the quality assurance umbrella of the European Committee on Breast Cancer Screening.

Delegations from the seven pilot studies met frequently in Brussels under the chairmanship of Monsieur Richonier from the European Commission. The External Advisers included Professor Fritz De Waard, from the Dom Project in Utrecht, and Dr Sven Törnberg, who was the co-ordinator of the screening programme in Stockholm, Sweden.

Guidelines were established for breast cancer screening and protocols agreed by all seven participating countries. It was agreed that annual audits would be carried out in individual countries by Professor De Waard on behalf of the European Commission.

Funding for breast cancer screening

The stimulus for the pilot screening programme was provided by funding from the European Action Against Breast Cancer Screening Committee. Total European funding over the four-year period was about £3 million (Irish pounds). This represented about 25% of the total funds necessary to carry out two rounds of screening. The remainder was raised by voluntary subscription through the Mater Foundation; Femscan, a voluntary organisation of women's groups (which raised over £150 000); the Department of Health, which made a contribution in the last two years of the screening programme; and the Irish Cancer Society, which funded a Nurse Counsellor.

The screening population

The decision in Brussels to screen women aged 50–65 in a population screening programme was adapted for use by the Eccles Breast Cancer Screening Programme. The catchment area was defined as North Dublin City, North Dublin County and the rural counties of Cavan and Monaghan. The total population was approximately 29 525. The screening interval was two years, and two view mammography was carried out on all women who accepted an invitation. In addition, supplemental X-rays such as paddle compression and Ultrasound were carried out where necessary.

In the first year of screening, the use of fine needle aspiration was introduced, modelled on the techniques developed at the Karolinska Clinic, Stockholm, in order to minimise the number of referrals for surgery.

Equipment and staff

The X-ray equipment was Mammot II, purchased from Siemens and installed in the static evaluating centre at 46 Eccles Street and in the Mobile Unit. The processing was Agfa Gevaert with a dedicated processing unit. The addition of stereotactic biopsy technology facilitated fine needle aspiration biopsy.

Parameters defined by the European Breast Cancer Screening Group were used to ensure Quality Control and these were applied by the Medical physics Department of the Diagnostic imaging Centre.

Staffing consisted of a Superintendent Radiographer, Miss Orla Laird, who was qualified as a teacher in Diagnostic Radiography and also had a Diploma in Mammography, four part-time Radiographers, two Secretaries and one Nurse Counsellor. In addition, there was one part-time Cytologist Technician and one part-time Cytopathologist, Dr Mary Dowling.

The Radiologists were interpreted by members of the Radiology Consultant group at the Mater Misericordiae Hospital. Despite several attempts, no suitably trained Radiologist could be obtained for the programme.

Conclusions

The Pilot Study demonstrated some important parameters that would help to establish a national screening programme in Ireland. The current prevalent rate of cancer was 7.9 per 1000. In the first round of screening, the recall rate was just over 4% and this dropped to 1.7% in the second round of screening. The benign to malignant biopsy ratio in the first round of screening was 1:1 and 0.4:1 in the second round of screening.

There was a marked reduction in the number of benign lesions referred for surgery in the second round of screening, due to the expertise which had been developed in fine needle aspiration and mammographic interpretation.

The overall effect of the Eccles Breast Cancer Screening Programme was to establish very important credential for the introduction of a national screening programme. This is currently being evaluated by the Department of Health.'

Professor J.T. Ennis, Institute of Radiological Sciences, Dublin, Ireland.

A short conclusion

There can be no doubt that funding is a powerful incentive to action, especially at a time when money is in short supply in the public sector. This is especially true of innovative and developmental stages of activities, which are most vulnerable to cuts and reductions in budgets because the viability or transferability of the work is unproven.

European funding has been the subject of much criticism, and numerous cases of fraudulent practices have occurred where there have been insufficient checks and policing of the system. There have also been instances where governments themselves have ignored or wilfully misunderstood principles such as that of additionality. Nevertheless, valuable developmental work has been undertaken and considerable transnational networking achieved for what is essentially a modest amount of money by national government standards. The Common Agricultural Policy remains the Achilles heel of the European Union, but apart from that, it is fair to say that EU funding represents good value for money. The efforts made by the European Commission to combat fraud unfortunately mean that many programmes will become more bureaucratic.

The major problem is really one of perception. The public are encouraged (at least here in the UK) to think about European Union membership in terms of money; money spent on support for agriculture, money levied on the British taxpayer to support European programmes, and money gained via European grants. Only comparatively recently have policy issues begun to feature regularly on the media scene, and these are still rare in the tabloid press. This superficiality of treatment means that tabloid newspaper readers (i.e. the majority of people who take a newspaper at all) are accustomed to forming their opinions on the basis of a superficial level of information, heavily biased, from sources which blatantly seek to manipulate.

The preoccupation with funding at the expense of policy issues is not merely regrettable, it is potentially damaging. In many institutions and public authorities, European funding is something of an obsession which may be allowed to obscure the really important issues. The scramble to secure funding under one programme or another often becomes a compelling activity in its own right which drains away valuable resources from other work. Some staff with a European brief may even be given targets relating to the level of income they must generate from EU-funded programmes.

There is nothing wrong with gaining and using funding from European programmes; in fact, it is an excellent way of focusing on an activity or proposed initiative and defining its aims and potential benefits. However, applicants must be putting forward proposals which have substance in their own right, and which are genuinely worthy in themselves. Ideally, they will be supportive of the organization's strategic plan and in line with European, national and local priorities – rather than being essentially a money-spinner for the organization concerned. There should be a clear and easily understandable relationship between a proposed activity for which funding is sought, and the European policy to which it relates.

Organizations themselves should also ensure that they promote a culture of European policy awareness and understanding, and that it is into this context that any exploitation of funded programmes fits. Strategic planning requires strategic thinking.

Summary points

1 After the Common Agricultural Policy, a large part of the EU's budget is spent on funding programmes which give substance to its policies. Funding for a variety of actions, usually on a partial basis, is accessible when a bidding organization can demonstrate congruence between its own objectives and Union policy.
2 Health care organizations should not simply try to fit into existing European programmes. They should also be actively influencing the Commission on future policy and helping to shape the thrust of future funding support.
3 Funding relevant to the health services fits into a framework of:
   • Structural funds – such as the European Regional

Development Fund (ERDF) and European Social Fund (ESF);

- Community initiatives like Horizon, Now, Adapt and Youthstart;
- Education and training programmes – Socrates and Leonardo da Vinci, which incorporate a number of earlier programmes such as Erasmus, Comett, Eurotecnet, Force, Lingua, Petra and Tempus;
- Research and Development, Fourth Framework Programmes – including the health-related programmes of Biotechnology, Biomedicine and Telematics for Health;
- specific health-related programmes covering health promotion, Europe Against Cancer, AIDS and other communicable diseases, and drugs.

4 Many (with the exception of the structural funds) require a transnational dimension involving partnership with organizations in other Member States.

References and further reading

Davison, A. (1993). *Grants from Europe: How to get money and influence policy*, 7th edn. NCVO, London.

Key data on education in the European Union, 1994. (1995). Office for official publications of the European Communities Task Force for Education, Training and Youth, European Commission.

These next two booklets are essentially reference documents rather than additional reading, but they cover the whole range of funded programmes in more depth than this chapter can. They are updated regularly, but obviously do not provide the detail necessary for making applications under the programmes themselves, and intending applicants should contact the appropriate unit dealing with the programme concerned as soon as possible. (Some contact names and addresses are provided in the Resource section.)

Sources of European Community Funding, 2nd edn. (1995). The Representation of the European Commission in the United Kingdom.

Finance from Europe. (A guide to grants and loans from the European Union.) (1995). Compiled for the Representation of the European Commission in the UK by Dr Michael Hopkins, Loughborough University Library. Produced in co-operation with the National Westminster Bank.

9

How to influence the European agenda

Aims of this Chapter

In this chapter, we aim to:
- explain the importance of influencing European policy and decision-making;
- discuss some of the relevant issues and problems;
- provide some pointers on how to do it;
- give an example of a lobbying organization and its aims.

The UK could and should exert progressive pressure for improvement in every area of EU policy, in the interests not just of Britain, but of Europe as a whole, and that's the EUROTRUTH.

The Right Honourable Neil Kinnock, European Commissioner for Transport. (From *Do you STILL believe all you read in the newspapers*, European Commission, 1995.)

European decision-making: somebody else's business?

Media coverage of the European Union, particularly since the Maastricht Treaty, has made people far more aware of the fact that decisions taken in Brussels and Strasbourg affect virtually every aspect of our daily lives. As well as influencing us as citizens and consumers, recent changes inspired by the European Union have almost certainly brought fresh challenges and new opportunities to the organizations in which we work or study. The European Union is now creating a new dynamism in many areas affecting the health systems and services of the Member States. The most obvious cases result from the 'four freedoms' – freedom of movement of goods, service, workers and capital – but European policies, as already explained, affect areas such as education, regional development, research and development, technology transfer and of crucial importance, public health itself. This breadth of activity requires an interactive and corporate approach within organizations, rather than a departmental one.

Organizations in the UK may currently seem a long way from what is known as 'the heart of the heart of Europe', yet we cannot ignore the plethora of policy documents, regulations, directives and decisions which emanate from the European Union, and which include a range of diverse issues relevant to the health sector, such as:

- health and safety at work;
- consumer protection;
- standards, for example in the areas of food law, environmental protection and pharmaceuticals;
- medical research;
- free movement of health professionals;
- health campaigns such as *Europe Against Cancer* and similar action against AIDS and communicable diseases;
- and the European Charter on Environment and Health (a WHO Charter endorsed by the European Union).

The role and powers of the European Union's institutions have been described in an earlier chapter. The European decision-making process is by no means simple and straightforward, and the policies and legislation which emerge rarely do so smoothly and easily. The fact is that the European Union is not a federation of like-minded states sharing a broadly similar culture, language and history. It is a diverse and rich collection of peoples and cultures with a history of interaction, sometimes benign, more often hostile, sharing a geographical base. The European institutions are committed to retaining and even supporting that diversity, including the retention of a number of languages. The European Union seeks to retain the richness of European culture but to forge an 'ever closer union' which will transcend the history of conflict and provide an enduring basis for peaceful co-operation.

Language – the ultimate barrier

Language is perhaps the most obvious of barriers to pan-European interaction at the level on which most ordinary people operate. Without fluency in the host language it is impossible to live and work in another country and most semi-skilled and unskilled workers throughout the EU are only proficient in their mother tongues. There are exceptions, however, and some countries have become almost polyglot, most notably the Dutch and Belgians. For the skilled worker, and for professionals and business people throughout the rest of the EU, fluency in at least one other European language – almost inevitably English – is becoming more usual. In the UK, it is a different matter; we have retained our insularity in terms of language competence and are depending more and more upon our fellow Europeans' command of English to communicate. Business people are catching on to the need for fluency in other languages but this is seen as a managerial issue rather than one for the shop floor.

It is interesting to speculate on whether we are witnessing the emergence of English as a new 'lingua franca', but at the same time the dangers of this must not be overlooked. Competence in a language enables communication in that language. If a Greek or Portuguese person wishes to initiate an interaction with a British colleague, the resultant conversation will almost certainly be in English. The British colleague may be comfortable with this, but effectively it means that the partnership is largely controlled by the other person, being established and maintained on their initiative. If a British organization wishes to undertake a European project, it will be forced to work with partners who speak English. Frustrations often arise over misunderstandings or lack of clarity, and this is exacerbated by extensive use of technical language and jargon.

No consultation without information

These barriers slow down progress in the whole range of European initiatives and developments. The 'Citizens Europe' dear to the hearts of those in the European Commission is simply a concept if the citizens concerned are unable to talk to each other. More importantly, if the decision-making process, including policy formation, is to be as open as possible, then all information must be accessible and available to Europe's citizens.

At the moment, most ordinary people are unaware that they have potential to influence European policy formation, other than via their own MP or MEP, and to a large extent this is mirrored in many organizations. It is particularly true of the public health sector; UK-based health care organizations need to challenge the insularity inherent in their systems and encourage their own staff to think more globally. Simply being kept informed about European developments is not enough; it is essential that health care organizations, and individual professionals, become more involved in influencing the direction of policy. There are also important implications for staff development and training programmes, as previously discussed; most of these continue to be placed within a national context and rarely include language acquisition or development.

Opening up the health debate

In all European countries, the future of public health is under debate. Decisions on health-related matters are increasingly being taken by national governments working together at a European level. Under the provisions of the Treaty on European Union (the Maastricht Treaty) the EU has a duty to plan a more active role in safeguarding our general health. Whilst it will not be able to intervene with the running of the NHS, the European Union will become increasingly influential in areas of our health that are linked, for example, to the environment or our behaviour.

There is likely to be more discussion at European level about just how far to proceed with EU action on health and health-related issues; suggestions have been made that national governments should maintain their grip on health matters or even tighten it, but it seems unlikely that this will ultimately be the case. Common sense dictates that if the 'ever-closer union' envisaged at Maastricht is to become a reality, over-arching policy decisions must be made at EU level and enforced in all Member States. The more purely national policies are formulated and implemented, the more confusion and lack of coherence there is likely to be, especially in areas where certain activities, such as drug misuse, are criminalized in one Member State and regarded as a health issue in another. Although European integration will not result in a single health care system, the closer relationship among member nations, and the members' desires for competitive advantage in the new market place, will lead to an interest, if not an imperative, in comparing health care systems along cost and quality dimensions.

The recent Andersen report, *The Future of European Health Care*, is an indicator of such moves.

Decisions taken in the European Union will continue to affect many areas related to both the providers and purchasers of health care. However, these decisions involve democratic processes, whether it is with regard to public health policy or any other area of European Union activity. Most health care professionals are aware of the mechanisms for consultation on national proposals, but are ignorant of European proposals and the channels of communication open to those wishing to influence them. This is something which tends to be left to the health departments of national governments, who can decide to carry out their own consultations, which may be limited in scope and involve only selected respondents. If practitioners or interest groups want to ensure that their concerns are taken into account, they must themselves take steps to be kept informed and to get involved with the decision-making process.

Making your voice heard

Those organizations which do not accept a passive role and are determined to influence policy formation at European level have decisions to take about their approach and degree of involvement. There are umbrella groups or interest groups which exist to represent the views and concerns of sectors, such as the European Public Health Alliance (which is described later in this chapter). Many organizations choose to operate through these, as they lack the resources or the inclination to mount their own lobbying campaigns. Others may choose to take independent action, perhaps on a specific issue which is of particular concern, such as a new piece of legislation in preparation.

According to the DTI publication *Brussels Can You Hear Me?* (DTI and Central Office of Information, 1993), there are five key points to follow for those who want to have their voice heard in Brussels. These are:

1 Get in early – there is a very clear process of decision-making in the European Union often involving many stages of consultation. Getting involved means doing so before formal drafts have been produced, if possible.
2 Work with others – a spread of opinion carries more weight than a lone voice. Networking, collaborating, forming partnerships, etc. are all vital requirements for organizations or individuals wanting to exert influence.
3 Think European – the European Union fosters the ideals of sharing, of working together to find common solutions to problems. To influence the Commission or any other European Union (EU) institution, ideas and or projects must serve to benefit the Community, not narrow protective interests.
4 Be prepared – try to find out what others think about a proposal. Be clear about what you or your organization want to achieve and be prepared to back up your case with the best available evidence.
5 Get involved – it is important to be plugged into the Brussels network in order to be able to react quickly to events as they arise.

This makes the whole process sound easy, though of course it is not. However, those involved in influencing decision-making at EU level do not do so alone. If they are acting as members of a pressure group or a professional association, this enables the burden to be shared and may assist with resource problems. Conversely, there is no reason why individuals cannot participate in the process and attempt to influence European legislation or actions, and in doing so would almost certainly meet like-minded people with whom they could join forces. (This is, after all, the way in which many pressure groups of long standing first began.) In fact, for every new policy area or item of legislation there is usually a plethora of different interests being brought to bear on the European institutions, and also on the national governments which will play their part in European decision-making.

How, and who, to target?

Careful targeting of those involved in policy formation and decision-making is essential, as is effective timing of all interventions. (The process was described in Chapter 3 and Figure 3 illustrates the process and charts the progress of legislation through the various institutions and stages of agreement.)

Individuals and organizations wishing to exert influence must first ensure that they are locked into the European information flow. The *Official Journal* and other documentation is widely available and approaches can also be made directly to Commission officials, MEPs and MPs, as well as national government officials. Policy documents are issued for consultation, often in various stages, and responses are welcomed from individuals as well as organizations. The key institutions include the following.

The European Commission

The national offices of the European Commission can provide general information and assistance, but the detailed work of the Commission takes place in Brussels and Luxembourg. Commission officials drafting policy documents and legislation are genuinely open to feedback, though this needs to be informed and clearly presented. It is also surprisingly easy to identify the individual officials involved, and their contact addresses and fax numbers. The Commission's Brussels offices are on various sites (especially since the refurbishment of the Berlaymont building forced staff to move out), but standard references like *Vacher's European Companion* (see Resource section) can help to pinpoint the relevant section within the DG concerned. If time is not a problem, the main Commission address (rue de la Loi 200, 1049 Brussels) can be used for preliminary enquiries.

Post-Maastricht, it was proposed that a key person would have responsibility for health matters within each Directorate General. These officials meet in an inter-departmental working group to ensure that public health matters are reflected in other European Union policies. The Commission also intends to set up a Health Protection Advisory Committee. The members, made up of three specialists from each Member State will meet twice a year to assess the pressing issues and study public health topics that the Commission plan to propose. The Committee would also help the Commission co-ordinate activities nationally and assist Member States to keep in contact with people in the business of applying the various public health initiatives.

DGV (Employment, Industrial Relations and Social Affairs) is taking the lead on implementation of the Public Health Article. New policy areas always entail a certain amount of fact finding on the part of the Commission initially, and the time to exert influence is always best when initiatives and policy-making are being developed, therefore contact with desk officers as well as policy-makers is an excellent strategy for those seeking to influence. Both the Europe Against AIDS and Europe Against Cancer programmes are organized via DGV, which has offices in both Brussels and in Luxembourg. (For information about other DGs with a health-related remit, see the European Commission factsheet in the Resource section of this book.)

In all dealings with the European Commission, it should be

borne in mind that staff are recruited from all Member States, some as secondees from Member State governments and some as Commission employees. It is likely that they will speak English, but this is not invariably the case, though those who do not speak English will certainly speak French as an alternative.

The European Parliament

As already indicated, the members of the European Parliament are attached to particular Committees. The remit of these Committees is to scrutinize the activities of both Commission and Council and to make amendments to proposals.

The main Committees which relate directly to health issues are:

- The Committee on the Environment, Public Health and Consumer Protection.
- The Committee on Social Affairs, Employment and Working Environment.
- The Committee on Culture, Youth, Education and the Media.

(The current UK membership of the Committee on the Environment, Public Health and Consumer Protection is listed in the European Parliament factsheet in the Resource section.)

Although MEPs divide a great deal of their time between Brussels and Strasbourg they also have local constituency offices which are always staffed in their absence. It is in the MEP's interests to understand local concerns and interests, and health care organizations should meet with, or at least have regular communication of some form with MEPs with health-related interests. They should also ensure that they have a good relationship with their own MEP.

The European Parliament also has an 'Intergroup' on public health. Intergroups are cross-party groups of MEPs, and though they have no legal status, they have an important role in enabling MEPs to interact with consumers, industry and interest groups. The Public Health Intergroup is chaired by Mel Read, MEP for Nottingham and Leicestershire North East, and she provides a brief account of its work below.

'The European Parliament's Public Health Intergroup was set up in 1993, in part because of the new Public Health Competence contained in the Maastricht Treaty. Members of the European Parliament from a broad political spectrum and from all 15 Member States now meet together in Strasbourg every month. To quote from the terms of reference, the group is intended to "provide MEPs with a forum to consider all aspects of public health policy within the European Union, and to represent European Union citizens' interests in the developing European Union public health agenda; especially in securing 'added value' of effective EU health protection policies".

However, the role of the European Parliament in public health matters predates the Intergroup, and indeed, the European Union has had an involvement in health matters since its inception.

The Union has been involved in a variety of environmental matters, on health and safety at work, on research, involving the Human Genome programme and diseases of socio-economic importance, consumer safety, telematics and health care and many other issues. A number of public health programmes on specific diseases have been set up, most notably the Europe Against Cancer Programme.

The Public Health Intergroup is both interested in and supportive of these initiatives and also of the Parliament's Environment and Public Health Committee. However, it is thought important that the Intergroup is not merely a reflection of the Committee, nor a passive commentator on European Union initiatives. For this reason, the Intergroup's terms of reference include "to consider how the totality of the European Union policies impact on health; in particular, to champion and monitor the implementation of Article 29 of the Maastricht Treaty, that 'health protection policies shall form a constituent part of the Community's other policies'".

Accordingly, the Intergroup was re-launched after the 1994 European Parliament elections, with an influx of new Members of diverse backgrounds and interests. Many came from the medical profession, including doctors and nurses, others from education, Trade Unions, community backgrounds or from consumer movements.

The programme of work reflected the diverse backgrounds of MEPs, and also the wish to consider many public health issues from a broad perspective. For example, the session on smoking and health included a presentation from a lawyer on tobacco products liability, a contribution from Europe Against Cancer, an overview of the European Parliament's initiatives on tobacco-related matters and presentations about tobacco control in France and Finland.

The session devoted to medicinal products gave the European Agency for the Evaluation of Medicinal Products, the pharmaceutical industry representatives, and BEUC (the European Consumers' Association) all an opportunity to contribute on this topic. The discussion drew out some key questions about patients' rights, about the role of drugs in medicine, about why and how people become ill in the first place and about the link between poverty and health.

The Intergroup has covered issues including drug addiction, the health of the elderly, contraception and sex education, blood product safety and the future development of the European Union Public Health Programme. A constant theme has been the need to draw into the discussion the views of consumers, who are rightly demanding more access to knowledge and influence. There is also a growing interest in the work of the Group, and requests to make presentations to the group from a wide range of organisations. Much of the credit for this must go to the European Health Alliance, whose professionalism in servicing the Group is a pivotal factor in its continuing success.

For the future, much depends on the ability of the Intergroup to continue to function completely independently of any commercial interests, and to attract a wide cross-section of Members of the European Parliament. There is likely to be an emphasis on particular policy areas combined with an appreciation that public health policy in the European Union must address a range of issues. Work, housing, income levels, environmental protection policies, consumer rights, research policies, agricultural practices, food policy, etc., all have major health implications.

Our final point in the terms of reference is "to seek open debate, and the widest possible consultation, in the development and introduction of action plans within the overall European Union Public Health programme".

A healthy Public Health Intergroup will hopefully have a significant part to play in future policy discussions.'

Mel Read, MEP.

The Economic and Social Committee (ECOSOC)

The main work of the ECOSOC is to deliver opinions on proposals for legislation issued by the Commission. Two of the nine ECOSOC sections deal with subjects of particular interest to health care.

1 The section for Protection of the Environment, Public Health and Consumer Protection.

2 The section for Social, Family, Educational and Cultural Affairs (which covers safety and health at work and occupational medicine).

Comments to draft proposals can be fed into these groups.

The 'social partners'

This phrase, unfamiliar to most British ears, refers to what is also known as 'the two sides of industry': that is, the employers and the unions. Involvement of the social partners at European level is perceived as essential, and UK involvement includes both the Confederation of British Industry (CBI) and the Trades Union Congress (TUC). These two groups are represented through the ECOSOC.

The Committee of the Regions

Established by the Treaty of European Union, the Committee's task was defined by Jacques Delors as a provider of democratic legitimacy to the EU. The intention was that by strengthening subsidiarity, working in tandem with the EP and giving a voice to citizens, the Committee would help to balance the 'democratic deficit', giving impetus to post-Maastricht Europe by communicating local concerns and grass-roots reactions and giving real substance to debates.

Public health is one of the Committee's special concerns. (The contact address of the Committee is provided in the Resource section.)

Influencing: a two-way process

As well as failing to influence the European Union, we often fail to be influenced by it. A great deal of developmental work is undertaken with support from the EU, and networks of demonstration projects have also been established. Many of these continue to be unknown and unappreciated, to some degree because insufficient attention is given to disseminating results (this is also a common failing of nationally based and funded work, too). One useful organization is the European Foundation for the Improvement of Living and Working Conditions (described in Chapter 5), which has managed or co-ordinated a series of projects and initiatives on issues relating to the quality of life and work, and disseminates information on these via its regular bulletins and annual reports. Many of the projects undertaken are of interest to health professionals.

Professional representation in the European Union

The European Commission has a highly developed system of internal consultation which is used to progress both policy development and implementation issues. The Commission encourages both formal and informal exchanges of information and expertise, in addition to supporting exchanges of personnel. It has also created various advisory and consultative groups which provide not only expert advice but can act as a channel of communication with practitioners in the field.

In cases where a professional group is covered by a specific sectoral directive (i.e. on recognition of professional qualifications), the Commission has also established Standing Advisory Committees. (In the case of the Professions Allied to Medicine (PAMs) which fall under the provisions of the UK Professions Supplementary to Medicine Act of 1960, no such groups currently exist at European level.)

Some health-related groups and standing committees

Various groups work with the Commission to provide expertise in specific professional areas and to represent the professional practice of the Member States. Membership of these groups is drawn from practitioners and recognized national experts, who themselves can act as a conduit for professional concerns and issues. The groups described below are a selection only rather than a complete list.

The Standing Committee of Nurses (PCN) was established in 1971, and is acknowledged by the Commission as the official liaison committee for the nursing profession. Membership is on the basis of one representative from each Member State, put forward collaboratively by the various national nursing associations. The Commission is bound to consult the Committee on relevant matters and the Committee can in turn present opinions and give advice to the Commission, as well as require information from its officials. The Committee has an office based in Brussels.

In 1979, the Council of Ministers decided to also set up the **Advisory Committee on Training in Nursing** (ACTN). One of a series of advisory groups (others include medical training and midwifery), its function is to advise the Commission on all aspects of nurse training and education. Members are proposed by national governments and appointed to the Committee by the Commission, and nominees, who serve for three years, are expected to contribute with a degree of objectivity as European professionals rather than as representatives of Member State interests. The UK currently has six representatives on the Committee.

The work of the Committee has moved through various phases. Initially it was concerned with assisting with the drafting of legislation to ensure a common standard of pre-registration level nurse training across the EC, and this was implemented during the 1980s. This applied to general nursing only and directives on paediatric and psychiatric nursing were not enacted. Now the approach has changed to one of harmonization, as already explained in Chapter 7, and the emphasis of the Committee's work has moved on to post-registration issues. The Committee's funding is tight, which has resulted in limitations in its workload, but new and valuable work is being undertaken nevertheless. Currently, work is underway on education and training for nurses caring for cancer patients and older people, and again the ACTN is aiming to assist the development of a consensual model to influence both pre- and post-registration training across the EU.

The Standing Committee of European Doctors was established in 1959, and was formerly called the Standing Committee of Doctors of the EC. Its membership is large compared with its counterpart committee for nurses, and British representation is via the British Medical Association (BMA). Its aims are to represent the medical profession of all the Member States, to study and promote high standards of medical practice and health care and to promote free movement of doctors. It also has an office based in Brussels.

The medical profession is also served by the **Advisory Committee on Medical Training**. This was set up in 1978, again with representatives selected by national governments on the advice of appropriate bodies. The BMA again provides the UK representation. Like the ACTN, this committee suffers from underfunding and the future of such groups may be in doubt.

Other professional groups in Europe

Various pan-European professional groups exist which were not established by the European Commission or supported by it, but are professional associations which have often developed from a practitioner base – for example, the European Union of Medical Specialists (EUMS), the European Federation of Professional Psychologists Associations, the European Nursing Group (ENG), and the European Association of Hospital Managers.

These groups are increasing rapidly and their variety and number make it difficult for the individual to assess how useful they can be, or how much influence they can exert on the European agenda. Undoubtedly many have the potential to be powerful forces for future consultation and for influencing policies at EU level, but they have the disadvantage of being outside the established circles set up by the European institutions for consultation purposes. These 'outsiders' have to prove themselves both to their membership and to the institutions they seek to influence. At the same time, the fact that they are practitioner- and profession-led, rather than government-sponsored, gives them a particular credibility of their own, and an accountability and allegiance to grass roots for any views they may express. This kind of independence might prove difficult for members of the Commission's Committees to sustain, should there be significant conflict between their professional views and national government thinking.

Presenting a united front

The health sector represents a multiplicity of interests. Yet whilst practitioners have different professional interests, they share common concerns, and these (though they may be viewed from a different perspective) are common to patients, their families and other interested individuals. One particularly effective way of influencing policy makers and decision makers has traditionally been by forming alliances with like-minded groups, or even banding together to adopt a broad spectrum approach. An example of such an approach is provided below.

Influencing the European health care agenda in practice: the European Public Health Alliance

Paul J. Belcher writes:
'Based in Brussels, the European Public Health Alliance (EPHA) is a non-profit making organisation comprised of non-governmental organisations in the health sector. Its primary tasks are to promote public health in Europe and to ensure participation of citizens in health-related policy-making. Since its formal launch in March 1993, EPHA has grown considerably, and currently represents almost 50 national and European organisations.

A voice for European citizens

There is a need for health associations to participate in discussion bearing on the future of health in the European Union. The success of the environmental movement demonstrates that Europeans understand the role of prevention and that they themselves wish to participate actively in the decisions made on their behalf.

Previously, consumers and patients have played only a very minor role in European policies affecting public health. The range of EU policies impacting on health has expanded over the years and it is now more important than ever to involve patients and consumers in the policy-making process. Public health now has a formal competence at EU level under Article 129 of the Treaty of European Union in areas such as prevention, information and education.

Membership

EPHA is open to non-profit-making associations independent of vested commercial interests from the following areas:

- associations concerned with health promotion and disease prevention;
- consumer and patient groups concerned with healthcare systems;
- disease specific groups representing the interests of sufferers and their families in relation to health scourges such as cardiovascular disease, cancer, AIDS, Alzheimer's, etc.;
- health and patient associations in the areas of mental and physical handicap;
- associations concerned with health-related issues such as tobacco, alcohol and narcotics;
- associations for which public health is a major consideration such as consumer, development and environmental organisations.

Activities

Advocacy   A central role of EPHA is to alert its members to important EU issues relevant to their specific interest, so that they can make their own approaches to European policy makers. The EPHA secretariat in Brussels provides the political support to facilitate such advocacy and maintains close contacts with policy makers in the European institutions. As well as informing members on their individual needs and interest, EPHA also concentrates on the more generic and long-term goals which are relevant to all member organisations and are in line with current EU public health initiatives. Some of the key demands made by EPHA are outlined below.

Health audit   All EU policy areas should be monitored constantly for their potential impact on health, in line with present arrangements for environmental impact assessment. Effective health audit has to be open and democratic, reflecting the commitment made in the Maastricht Treaty that "Health protection requirements shall form a constituent part of the Community's other policies".

An overall health programme   A more coherent strategy is needed, not fragmented among several Directorates General.

A European Commissioner for Health One Commissioner should assume responsibility for all EU public health activities.

Pushing health up the political agenda Health should receive the same political attention that is now given to environmental issues.

Adequate finance and staffing for health The budgetary allocation for activities relating to public health should be greatly increased and better resources are needed for the public health unit of DGV of the European Commission.

Defending health at the 1996 Inter-governmental Conference The existing health competence should be maintained and extended at next year's IGC.

Patients' rights The Commission should take into account patients' rights in a wide context other than simply as users of health services.

Information service

EPHA provides an information service which monitors EU health policy development on a daily basis. In addition to responding to queries from the general public, MEPs and NGOs (Non-governmental organisations), the monthly EPHA bulletin "European Public Health Update", aims to inform readers of health activities in the European Union.

1995 Public Health Hotline

In order to increase awareness of the new EU competence in public health, to inform the public of the EU's actions in this field, and to canvass public opinion on how EU public health might develop, EPHA organised a Public Health Hotline in May 1995, with financial support from the European Commission. Community-wide press coverage was arranged prior and during the event and a series of 13 briefing papers were produced on different aspects of European policies that affect public health. These have now been published in book form. The results of the week-long event were presented to the Commission and the Health Intergroup of the European Parliament. The Hotline highlighted the need for routine and easily-accessible information. EPHA is now working towards providing a permanent and independent EU public health information service.

Intergroup on Health at the European Parliament

EPHA provides the secretariat for the Intergroup on Health at the European Parliament. The Intergroup meets during the plenary session of the European Parliament in Strasbourg and provides an open forum for policy-makers and interested groups to exchange views with MEPs on pertinent issues related to public health. In 1995, Intergroup meetings have been held on tobacco and health, development of an EU health policy, the fight against drug abuse, the European Medicines Evaluation Agency, and the elderly and mental illness. Other Intergroup meetings are planned for later this year on sex education and contraception, and blood products. Possible topics for future meetings include health and the Inter-Governmental Conference, poverty and health, and alcohol.

Conferences

A number of European conferences have been organised by EPHA, with the support of the European Commission on a range of health issues. In recent years these have included: "Research Priorities for Public Health in Europe", "Social Inequalities and Health" (joint conference with the BMA and BMJ), and a major EU seminar on the "Future Development of EU Public Health Policy" held in 1994 in Limelette, Belgium. EPHA also provided the organisational support for the User and Industry Roundtable on Implementation of the Information Society in Health Care at a European Commission telematics conference held in Lisbon in December 1994. Possible topics for future conferences include patients' rights and health data and indicators.

The future of EU health activities

The Treaty on European Union is to be revised at the 1996 Inter-Governmental Conference and the European public health alliance would like to see both an extension of the EU's existing, limited competence in public health and better use of existing provisions.

Much more could be achieved within the existing provisions of Article 129 if greater political will had been demonstrated. Indeed, Padraig Flynn, European Commissioner with responsibility for health, has said that Article 129 is not yet fully understood as Member States continue to view EU action as a threat to national sovereignty. This has resulted in too much emphasis being put on the "risks" of action rather than the "opportunities". As well as calling for better implementation of Article 129, EPHA also calls for a clearer legal base to permit greater EU action on health rather than solely co-ordination, as is currently the case.

Article 129 is being interpreted in various ways by Member States. Some states consider that EU responsibility in disease prevention should be confined to health information and education. EPHA is opposed to such a restrictive "minimalist" definition and calls for prevention to be interpreted in the broadest sense, incorporating topics such as the exchange of experience in cancer care, the rehabilitation of drug addicts and combating discrimination against AIDS patients.

National governments are, however, keen to protect their power and it is unclear just how far they will go in asserting the principle of subsidiarity to minimise future EU competence in the field of public health. Unfortunately, disease and poor health have little respect for national sovereignty and pose great challenges throughout all member states – such as the ageing of populations, increasing numbers of AIDS and drug abuse cases, and increasing mobility of people within the EU and the subsequent spread of communicable diseases and illegal drugs. Improving the health of all EU citizens requires determined action at European as well as national level. As Mrs Simone Veil, former President of the EU Health Council, said in her address to the European Parliament's Committee on the Environment, Public Health, and Consumer Protection, on 23 January 1995: "... if we want to bring the EU closer to our citizens, we certainly should consider public health as an EU responsibility".'

Paul J. Belcher

Other umbrella organizations are adopting a similar approach, and networking with similar groups to form strategic alliances. One such group is Eurolink Age, which aims to represent and safeguard the interests of older people, and has close links with Age Concern.

Conclusions

The degree to which organizations become actively involved in influencing European policy or decision-making is obviously a decision for them alone to make. But at the very least, due consideration should be given to the *potential* for influencing, probably as part of the strategic planning process. It would appear that too much strategic planning is being done within a purely national context and that any European involvement or activity is frequently viewed as income-generational, or marginal, rather than policy-related and relevant to the whole organization.

Amongst the problems facing would-be 'influencers' in the UK is the fact that health here has become a highly politicized issue. The NHS itself is invariably caught up in a tug of war during every general election, with each political party trying to use it to assume moral superiority. Health issues are also used emotively, and are treated in this way frequently in the tabloid press.

One result appears to be that central government officials and politicians are extremely sensitive about health-related issues and feel threatened if they think that UK-based organizations are developing direct links with EU institutions. This is mild paranoia, because, as this book makes plain, the European institutions have very little actual power over health systems in member countries; the EU involvement in public health is complementary to work undertaken in Member States and subject to the principle of subsidiarity. Nevertheless, feedback from several sources indicates a reluctance on the part of the UK Department of Health to facilitate direct links between health trusts and EU institutions. All the more reason to refuse to play a passive role in the future of the European Union's public health policy and assume an active one instead!

Summary points

1 If European citizenship is to become more than a concept, people from different Member States must be able to talk to each other. If the EU's decision-making processes are to be open, then information must be accessible and available to Europe's citizens.

2 Simply being kept informed about European developments is not enough. Health care organizations are not fully exercising their capacity to influence European policy formation. Too much strategic planning is being done within a purely national context, with any European involvement frequently viewed as income-generational or marginal, rather than policy-related and relevant to the whole organization. They need to challenge the insularity inherent in their systems and encourage their staff to think more globally and become involved in influencing policy direction. If they do not, then the initiative will continue to rest restrictively with the health departments of national governments.

3 There are five key points to be observed in getting heard in

Brussels: get in early, work with others, think European, be prepared and get involved.

4 Careful targeting and timing are essential. First, individuals and organizations seeking to exert influence must ensure that they are locked into the European information flow through points of contact with the Commission, the Parliament, the committee system and health-related specialist groups.

5 As well as failing to influence the EU, we often fail to be influenced by it. A great deal of the development work undertaken on behalf of the Union continues to be unknown and unappreciated because of insufficient attention to dissemination. Improvements to the information flow are being helped by the work of organizations such as the European Foundation for the Improvement of Living and Working Conditions and the European Public Health Alliance.

References and further reading

Brussels Can You Hear Me? (1993) (How to influence the decision-making process). DTI Single Market publication (free), Central Office of Information, also a 13 minute video of the same title (£24.99).

Mazey, S. and Richardson, J. (eds) (1993). *Lobbying in the European Community*. Nuffield European Series, Oxford University Press.

10

A European Commission perspective

Padraig Flynn, European Commissioner with responsibility for health, answers questions on the EU's health care policies. (Note: At the time of writing, the European health programmes referred to by the Commissioner were still awaiting final approval.)

The EU's role in relation to health is largely perceived as confined to health protection and positive health promotion. Yet most people have a negative or 'deficit' view of health – in other words, they think of health services as services for unwell people and usually access them only when they are poorly. The Commission wants to promote the idea of well-being and positive health. How will this be done?

To begin with, I would like to clarify the EU's health role. It is not just confined to health protection and positive health promotion, as is commonly assumed. Our work is much broader. To name but a few matters, it includes environmental issues, food safety, development and emergency aid, research and development, the recognition of medical qualification and health and safety at work.

Nevertheless, I fully accept that the EU's most *visible* role is in relation to health protection and positive health promotion. As you rightly point out, most people only access the health services when they are ill. Unfortunately, individuals and health services have been far too slow to make preventative action more effective. It may be a cliché, but in relation to medical health, a stitch in time saves nine. In the EU today, the main causes of death are no longer infectious diseases but cardiovascular diseases, cancers, accidents and suicides. Habits and lifestyles are the major influences on those factors. We must promote healthier lifestyles, therefore, if we are to reduce the mortality and morbidity associated with these diseases. Simply put, if people eat better, exercise more and avoid certain known risk factors such as smoking, there would be tremendous improvements in health.

The Commission's efforts to promote a more positive health prevention message are focused on its health programmes. The programme for health information, education and training in particular aims to encourage the adoption of lifestyles conducive to better health. The other programmes currently before the Council and the European Parliament – on AIDS and other communicable diseases; on cancer; and on drug dependency – also contain a very important element on lifestyles. A clear emphasis in the cancer programme, naturally, is the need to quit smoking. Similarly in relation to the AIDS programme, there is a clear need to avoid risk factors, such as unsafe sex.

Do you think that Article 129 of the Maastricht Treaty goes far enough towards improving the health of Europe's citizens? In view of the next inter-govern-mental conference in 1996, would you welcome any changes in the Public Health Article?

Article 129 serves as a legislative base for the EU's action in the field of public health. It represented a major breakthrough, as prior to its adoption, the EU had limited competence in this area. It now has a clear mandate for action. As regards whether it goes far enough, time will be the judge. However, I think it is important to emphasize that legislation in itself is not the solution to public health problems – if it were, we would have legislated for the abolition of a host of public health problems a long time ago. What is important, is the effectiveness of the actions carried out under the legislation.

My priority, therefore, is to ensure that the action programmes which the Commission has proposed under

Article 129 are effectively implemented. To date, the Commission has tabled four such programmes: on cancer; AIDS and other transmissible diseases; health information training and education and, finally, on drug dependency. A fifth programme, on health data indicators, should be transmitted to the Council and European Parliament shortly. Meanwhile we are working on three further programmes in relation to accidents and injuries, pollution-related diseases and rare diseases.

This is an ambitious and wide-ranging series of programmes and is indicative of the wide scope which Article 129 gives the Commission. I might add that I am happy with the scope which Article 129 provides us in the public health area. As to whether the next IGC should consider changes, I believe similarly that it is too early to say. For the moment, I think it is far more important that the Commission gets on with effectively implementing its current health programmes rather than engaging in debate on extra powers or competences.

Article 129 requires that the Commission takes account of the health dimension of its other policies. Can you explain how this is achieved and what happens in practice?

Health considerations have always been a constituent part of overall Community policies. Apart from Article 129, health features in several key respects in the Union Treaty. For example, one of the key Treaty objectives, provided for in Article 2, is the 'raising of the standard of living and quality of life'. This involves clear health considerations. Similarly, other provisions of the Treaty deal with health standards in animal and vegetable products, health and safety at work and health factors in relation to the environment and consumer protection.

Under Article 129, the health role is, however, much more focused. It specifically requires 'that health protection requirements shall form a constituent part of the Community's other policies'. There is now an inter-service committee in the European Commission which deals with the implementation of this requirement. In practice, this entails looking at the full range of EU activities from a health viewpoint. Where specific issues arise, this in turn can lead to specialist inter-service committees such as on pharmaceuticals and public health.

The committee is also instrumental in the preparation of an annual report which provides information on the health implications of other policies. The first such report was approved by the Commission earlier this year and transmitted to the European Parliament and the Council. I emphasize that this is the first such report. Future reports will develop and improve on the first report and take into account the views of relevant bodies such as the Council and Parliament in this respect. I expect that the report will be discussed at the next Health Council scheduled for 30 November 1995. I am looking forward to hearing its views on the direction in which future reports should go.

There are many differences in attitudes, expectations and services of health and illness in Europe. Do you envisage a time when there will be a certain amount of convergence? If so, what do you see as the most likely areas for convergence?

There is already a growing amount of convergence. This is to be expected and encouraged, as clearly the ultimate objective must be to converge towards the best standards and practices.

The convergence is taking place from two directions. Firstly, health professionals are increasingly aware of medical and health care practices in other Member States. This is a process which the Commission actively encourages in its health programmes. Secondly – and of increasing importance – consumers are also much more aware and conscious of standards and practices elsewhere. If these are considered inadequate in their own country, questions and pressure for remedial action naturally arise.

I would cite breast cancer screening as an example. The extent and nature of screening differs substantially between Member States. This has led to pressure in Member States where the level of screening is minimal for increased resources to be allocated, so as to match the standards available in other

Member States. There was a similar experience in relation to issues such as operations for hip replacements, where waiting lists vary substantially between Member States.

I believe that convergence will continue in the above directions. I might add that the Commission has no proposals or competence to *require* such convergence. Article 129, for example, specifically excludes 'the harmonization of the laws and regulations of the Member States' from measures to be proposed under that Article. It is for each Member State to decide for itself how to organize and finance its health service and I do not challenge that right. However, the Commission does encourage co-operation between the Member States. A major initiative in this respect is the proposed health data indicators programme, which aims to make available a very wide range of comparable data relevant to the health area. This, in turn, will aid discussion and analysis of the state of health and the health services in the various Member States.

UK health and social organizations and the personnel working within them generally know very little about those EU policies and programmes which have most potential impact and opportunities for them. How do you think this can be addressed by the Commission or by others?

We are taking a number of steps to address this issue. In the overall context of the Commission's communications strategy, we are in the process of strengthening our capacity in this area and, for example, developing new materials about our work, such as a regular newsletter which will have a wide distribution. Our programmes are also putting an emphasis on information and outreach: for instance, through the activities undertaken in the context of the European weeks against cancer and against drugs, the presentations of some of the major AIDS projects at international conferences, and the development of the European Health-Promoting Schools Network. Another significant measure, which I referred to earlier, is our recent publication of the first report of the state of health in the European Community. This report sets out the major health trends in the Community and should help to make the reasons behind specific Community public health actions and their impact more visible to European citizens.

Beside the Commission, a number of other organizations are making efforts to improve the public's knowledge about, and understanding of, the Commission's work in this field. The European Public Health Alliance, for example, recently set up a telephone hotline on health, with our financial support, as a way of ascertaining the major concerns of the public and providing them with information on what the Community was doing in response. The European Healthcare Management Association is about to begin another project supported by us, which will investigate the practical problems people have when they move from country to country in obtaining the health services they need. They will also suggest ways in which these could be tackled by the Community.

Despite both sectoral and general systems directives, there has been very little professional mobility across Europe in the health and social sectors. In view of the demographic problems and areas of under/over supply in certain professional groups, how serious is this situation and what suggestions have you for increasing mobility?

Free movement of people is a major objective of the EU, enshrined in the Treaty. The Commission regards the promotion of professional mobility as an important aspect of its activities towards creating a single market.

The numbers of people moving from one Member State to another are rather low in most professions, not just in the health and social sectors. In fact, the situation in many health professions is relatively advantageous. A large number of legal obstacles to free movement have been removed by the sectoral Council directives and most professionals in this field could work in other countries without major adaptations or additional training being required. In countries where there is a specific demand for health care professionals, cross-border movement has increased.

That being said, when considering the numbers involved one should not forget that there are important cultural barriers to movement which are difficult to overcome, not least the question of languages. The Commission can only attempt to abolish existing barriers, but cannot obviously oblige people to exercise their right of free movement. Through a number of advisory committees for the different major professions as well as by means of regular contacts with professional organizations, the Commission is trying to identify the remaining problems and barriers to free movement and possibilities for overcoming them.

How important do you think it is that education and training for health and social care professionals has a European dimension?

Health and social care professionals are, in future, likely to come into contact with more and more clients originating in other Member States. In view of that, and also in order to enable and encourage professionals to exercise their right of free movement, it is important that their education and training take into account a European dimension. One important way of pursuing this objective is through the organization of personnel exchanges, which could be supported by the EU action programmes Socrates and Leonardo.

The European credit transfer system (ECTS), which is part of the Erasmus programme, includes, for example, possibilities for credit transfers of medical students. However, even if the number of exchanges rises considerably in the future, it is probable that only a minority of students will be involved. It is therefore also important to include a European dimension in the regular education and training curricula of health and social care professionals.

Europe's health and social care professions represent a huge number of people. Do you think that they could potentially become a forceful group, capable of influencing EU decisions, and if so, in what ways can they have a strong voice in Brussels?

Health and social care professionals do indeed constitute a large group of people in the European Community. But it is hard to see them acting as one unified group in the

Community, particularly since they do not do so at national or even local level.

However, individual professions and groups of professionals have set up bodies at European level to represent their interests and convey their views, and these are already playing an important role in the Community decision-making process. There is a growing number of such Community-wide organizations, which disseminate information, undertake educational activities, bring people together to exchange ideas, contribute to ongoing debates, and try to ensure that their views and concerns are taken into account when Community proposals are being formulated and decided upon.

Some of these organizations are based upon a particular profession, such as the Standing Committees of Nurses and of Doctors, or groups of professions, such as the Hospital Committee of the European Community (HOPE) and the European Healthcare Management Association. Others come together around a particular issue, such as the European Heart Network and EuroCASO, which groups together non-governmental organizations in the field of HIV and AIDS, or to promote more general aims, such as the European Public Health Alliance. Finally, a number of individual national organizations, such as the British Medical Association and the Swedish Institute for Health Services Development, also devote some energy to keeping abreast of what is happening in the Community and making an input where possible.

The public health programmes that we are developing provide for the establishment of advisory committees of representatives of the Member States. It is for the Member States to decide on their committee representatives. However, we have made it clear that we hope that the composition of these committees will ensure adequate representation of the interests and expertise of health professionals (in the widest sense) and non-governmental organizations as well as the national authorities.

Health and social networks in Europe, including professional, managerial and organizational, are currently somewhat unsophisticated. How would you like

to see more effective networks emerge and how can EU programmes assist this process?

As public health and health in general become firmly established as Community activities, and as the visibility of our actions grows, there seems little doubt that the health and social care professions will further increase the attention they pay to the Community. One obvious way to do this is to establish pan-Community organizations and networks that are able to address issues from a Community-wide perspective.

The development of interchanges between organizations is a major element of our public health strategy. Such networks provide a key mechanism for the exchange of ideas, experience and information and the spread of good practice, and can help to bridge the gap between the Community institutions and the general public.

In the light of this, the Commission provides financial support for the establishment and strengthening of a number of the health and social networks and for particular projects that they wish to undertake in the framework of the various Community programmes. In this way, the networks can make a direct contribution to the implementation of our activities, while at the same time developing our own work and strengthening their own organizational capabilities.

The EU funds a wide range of project work relevant to health and social care workers. Can you give examples of the type of projects you would be likely to support and the criteria for selection?

To implement our public health programmes, we employ several kinds of action. Our Communication of November 1993 on the *framework for action in the field of public health* set out the principal ones: the establishment of networks, the exchange of information and experience, the exchange of personnel, training, research and evaluation, programmes of information and education, and co-operative actions with other countries and international organizations.

The projects we support fall within these broad areas of work. We receive many more applications for support than we can fund. In deciding between them the key criterion that we use is whether they can demonstrate that they provide real added value for the European Community. To meet this criterion, a project should involve the participation of at least two Community Member States, or be conducted jointly in several Member States. Projects relating to only one Member State may also be supported, however, where they are innovative activities which can be used as a model by other Community Member States, or which will provide information of use to them.

Another important criterion, is that in line with Article 129 of the EU Treaty, public health projects should be primarily related to the main focus of our work which is on prevention and health promotion, rather than to care and treatment. Health and social care workers should, therefore, put the emphasis on those elements in any projects they put forward.

Resource section

This section contains material in support of earlier chapters and includes information on the European Commission and Parliament, useful contacts and organizations and a glossary of terms. *Although every effort has been made to ensure that these details were accurate at the time the book went to press, things can change very quickly on the European scene, and it would be wise to anticipate this and not expect information to remain current for long periods.*

Resource section contents

Part 1 Factsheets on the European Commission and Parliament
Part 2 Useful contacts and sources of information
Part 3 Select glossary of terms and 'Eurojargon'

Part 1

Factsheet 1 Commission of the European Communities (CEC)

The Commission is based in Brussels, with 24 Directorates General overseen by 20 Commissioners from 15 Member States.

Its official Brussels address is:

Commission of the European Communities
200 Rue de la Loi
1049-Brussels
Belgium
Tel. 00 322 2991111

(Addresses for UK offices can be found in Part 2, in the 'contacts' list.)

The Commissioners

The members of the current Commission, with their responsibilities, are as follows:

Jacques Santer (Luxembourg)
President of the Commission
Responsible for the Secretariat-General, the Legal Service, Security Office, Forward Studies Unit, Inspectorate General, Joint Interpreting and Conference Service, Monetary matters (with M Silguy), Institutional issues and Intergovernmental Conference (with Mr Oreja) and Common Foreign and Security Policy (with Commissioner van den Broek).

Martin Bangemann (Germany)
Industrial Affairs; Information Technologies and Telecommunications.

Ritt Bjerregaard (Denmark)
Environment; Nuclear Safety.

Emma Bonino (Italy)
Fisheries; Consumer Policy; European Community Humanitarian Office.

Sir Leon Brittan (UK)
External relations with North America, Australia, New Zealand, Japan, China, South Korea, Hong Kong, Macao, Taiwan; Common Commercial Policy; Relations with OECD and WTO.

Hans van den Broek (Netherlands)
External relations with Central and Eastern Europe and former Soviet Union, Turkey, Cyprus, Malta, other European countries; Common Foreign and Security Policy; External Service.

Edith Cresson (France)
Science, Research and Development; Joint Research Centre; Human Resources, Education, Training and Youth.

Joao de Deus Pinheiro (Portugal)
External Relations with the countries of Africa, Caribbean and Pacific; South Africa, Lomé Convention.

Franz Fischler (Austria)
Agriculture and Rural Development.

Padraig Flynn (Ireland)
Employment and Social Affairs; Relations with the Economic and Social Committee.

Anita Gradin (Sweden)
Issues relating to home affairs, judiciary and immigration; relations with the European Ombudsman; Anti-fraud measures, Financial Control.

Neil Kinnock (UK)
Transport.

Erkki Liikanen (Finland)
Budget; Personnel and Administration; Translation and Information Technology.

Manuel Marin (Spain)
External Relations with the (Southern) Mediterranean,

Middle and Near East, Latin America and Asia (excluding areas covered by Leon Brittan).

Karel Van Miert (Belgium)
Competition.

Mario Monti (Italy)
Internal Market; Financial Services; Customs and Indirect Taxation; Direct Taxation.

Marcelino Oreja (Spain)
Relations with the European Parliament; Relations with the Member States on openness, communication and information; Culture and Audiovisual; Publications Office; Institutional questions; preparation for the 1996 IGC (with the Presidency).

Christos Papoutsis (Greece)
Energy and Euratom Supply Agency; Small and Medium sized Enterprises (SMEs); Tourism.

Yves-Thibault de Silguy (France)
Economic and Financial Affairs; Monetary matters (with the Presidency); Credit and Investments; Direct Taxation.

Monika Wulf-Mathies (Germany)
Regional Policies; Relations with the Committee of the Regions; the Cohesion Fund (in agreement with Commissioners Kinnock and Bjerregaard).

Each Commissioner has a *cabinet* (pronounced in the French way) of his/her own staff.

The Directorates General

The work of the Commission is divided between the DGs, and supported by other units such as the Security Office, the Translation Service, the Statistical Office (EUROSTAT), the Legal Service and others. The Secretariat-General of the Commission manages its interactions with the other institutions plus internal co-ordination and planning. In addition, there are other agencies or organizations which are part of the Commission, such as the European Community Humanitarian Office (ECHO), the Office for Official Publications, the European Foundation for the Improvement of Living and

Working Conditions and the European Centre for the Development of Vocational training (CEDEFOP).

The DGs themselves are as follows:

DGI	External Economic Relations
DGIA	External relations: Europe and the New Independent States, common foreign and security policy and external missions
TFE	The Enlargement Task Force
DGII	Economic and Financial Affairs
DGIII	Industry
DGIV	Competition
DGV	Employment, Industrial and Social Affairs
DGVI	Agriculture
	Veterinary and Phytosanitary Office
DGVII	Transport
DGVIII	Development
DGIX	Personnel and Administration
DGX	Information, Communication Culture and Audio-visual
DGXI	Environment, Nuclear Safety and Civil Protection
DGXII	Science, Research and Development
	Joint Research Centre
DGXIII	Telecommunications, Information Market and Exploitation of Results
DGXIV	Fisheries
DGXV	Internal Market and Financial Services
DGXVI	Regional Policy and Cohesion
DGXVII	Energy
DGXVIII	Credit and Investments
DGXIX	Budgets
DGXX	Financial Control
DGXXI	Customs and Indirect Taxation
DGXXII	Education, Training and Youth
DGXIII	Enterprise policy, Distributive Trades, Tourism and Co-operatives
DGXIV	Consumer policy

European Commission sections/contacts responsible for health-related matters and other areas of interest

Human Resources and Networks
DGXXII   Education, Training and Youth
Mutual Recognition of Professional Qualifications – regulated professions
DGXV/E/2   Jacqueline Minor or Jean-Marie Visée
Equal Opportunities between men and women
DGV/A/3   Agnes Hubert
Ethnic minorities ('migrant workers')
DGV/D/3   Rob Cornelissen
Disabled people
DG V/E/3   Bernhard Wehrens
Relations with WHO and other international organizations
DGI
Consumer goods (including food products, biotechnology and relationship between diet and health)
DGIII/E
Health and safety at work
Occupational accidents and injuries
DGV/F/4   Ramon Biosca de Sagastuy
Occupational health and hygiene
DGV/F/5   Ronald Haigh
Public health
(Policy and programme co-ordination, public health analysis)
DGV/F/1   Georges Gouvras
Disease-specific programmes
DGV/F/2   Yves Morettini
Europe Against Cancer
DGV/F/2   Soledad Blanco Mangudo
Health promotion and disease surveillance
DGV/F/3
Agriculture and health
DGVI/B/II
Telematics for health
DGXIII/C/4
Telematics for the elderly and disabled
DGXIII/C/5   Egidio Ballabio

Nuclear safety
DGXI/C//4 (civil protection)   A. Barisch
DGXII/F/6 (Radiation protection and biological effects)
              Kenneth Chadwick
Life sciences and technologies
DGXII/E/4 Medical research   André Baert
Pharmaceuticals
DGIII/E/3   Patrick De Boyser

(See the contacts list for details of European-funded programme contacts.)

Factsheet 2

The European Parliament

Parliament is the major democratic institution of the EU, being the only directly elected body. (The Committee of the Regions is made up of previously elected representatives from local and regional authorities, rather than people who have been directly elected to the Committee.) It represents 370 million people in total, and Euro-constituencies tend to be much larger than national government constituencies.

The Member States were sensitive about the location of the European institutions. There is a new, purpose-built Parliament building in Brussels but plenary sessions are still held in Strasbourg one week each month, though Committees and several other meetings take place in Brussels, which is obviously more convenient for close contacts with the Commission and the Council. The Secretariat is in Luxembourg. This fragmenting of centres means that MEPs and staff travel a great deal, which results in extra costs and less time spent in their constituencies.

The addresses of the European Parliament are as follows:

Secretariat:
European Parliament
L-2929 Luxembourg
Tel 0035243001

Strasbourg:
Palais de l'Europe
F-67006
Strasbourg Cedex
France
Tel 00 33 88174001
Fax 00 33 256501

Brussels:
97–113 Rue Belliard
B-1047 Brussels
Belgium
Tel 00 322 2842111
Fax 00 322 2846933

The European Parliament now comprises 626 members. The breakdown is as follows:

Germany	99	Portugal	25
France	87	Sweden	22
Italy	87	Austria	21
UK	87	Denmark	16
Spain	64	Finland	16
Netherlands	31	Ireland	15
Belgium	25	Luxembourg	6
Greece	25		

Parliament has a President, Klaus Hänsch, with 14 Vice Presidents assisting him. Members sit together in the chamber according to their political groupings. The largest group is the party of European Socialists, with 221 seats (chaired by Pauline Green).

Committees

Standing Committees of the Parliament do the detailed work necessary before issues can be discussed and agreed in plenary session (a list of the Committees was provided in Chapter 3).

The Committee on the Environment, Public Health and Consumer Protection (C11) is of most interest to health care professionals. Its UK membership is as follows:

- Ken Collins   Chair
  MEP for Strathclyde East
- Caroline Jackson   Vice Chair
  MEP for Wiltshire North and Bath
- David Bowe
  MEP for Cleveland and Richmond
- Anita Pollock
  MEP for London South West
- Susan Waddington
  MEP for Leicester
- Ian White
  MEP for Bristol

- Phillip Whitehead
  MEP for Staffordshire East and Derby

(A full list of UK MEPs and their constituencies is available from the UK European Parliament office in London. See the 'contacts' list for the address.)

Part 2

Useful contacts and sources of information

Section A   International, European and national contacts –
general and health care interest

Section B   Contacts for European programmes

Section C   Information networks: European Documentation
Centres, Euro Info Centres and EURES Euroadvisers in the UK

Section D   Useful publications (including on-line information)

Section A International, European and national contacts – general and health care interest

1. International and European institutions and organizations

European Parliament

Palais de l'Europe
F-67006 Strasbourg Cedex
France
Tel 00 33 88 174001
Fax 00 33 88 256501

Rue Belliard 97–113B
B-1047 Brussels
Belgium
Tel 00 32 2 284 2111
Fax 00 32 2 284 6933

L-2929 Luxembourg
Tel 00 352 43001
Fax 00 352 43 40 72

UK information point

European Parliament UK Office
2 Queen Anne's Gate
London SW1H 9AA
Tel 0171 222 0411
Fax 0171 222 2713
Head: Martyn Bond   Deputy Head: John Horton

(See the factsheet for more information.)

European Commission

Headquarters (postal address for whole Commission)

Commission of the European Communities
Rue de la Loi 200
B-1049 Brussels
Belgium
Tel 00 322 2991111

(See the CEC Factsheet for a list of Directorates General and other information.)

UK offices
Jean Monnet House
8 Storey's Gate
London SW19 3AT
Tel 0171 973 1992
Fax 0171 973 1900
Head of the Representation: Geoffrey Martin

Northern Ireland
Windsor House
9/15 Bedford Street
Belfast BT2 7EG
Tel 01232 240708
Fax 01232 248241
Head of Office: Jane Morrice

Wales
4 Cathedral Road
Cardiff CF1 9SG
Tel 01222 371631
Fax 01222 395489
Head of the Representation: Jorgen Hansen

Scotland
9 Alva Street
Edinburgh EH2 4PH
Tel 0131 2252058
Fax 0131 2264105

Economic and Social Committee

2 Rue Ravenstein
B-1000
Brussels
Belgium
Tel 00 322 5469011
Fax 00 322 5134893

The Committee of the Regions

2 Rue Ravenstein

B-1000 Brussels,
Belgium
Tel 00322 546 2211
Fax 00322 546 2085

Statistical Office (EUROSTAT)

Batiment Jean Monnet
Rue Alcide de Gasperi
L-2920 Luxembourg
Tel 00 352 43011 33107
Fax 00 352 4301 33015

European Agency for the Evaluation of Medicinal Products

7 Westferry Circus
Canary Wharf
London E14 4HB
Tel 0171 418 8400
Fax 0171 418 8416

Agency for Health and Safety at Work

Bilbao, Spain (address not yet available)

European Monitoring Centre for Drugs and Drug Addiction

Temporary address: Centro Luxor
76 Rua da Misericordia
1200 Lisbon
Portugal

Court of Justice of the European Communities

Palais de la Cour de Justice
L-2925 Luxembourg

European Free Trade Association (EFTA)

9–11 Rue de Varembé
CH 1211
Geneve 20
Switzerland

Tel 00 41 227491111
Fax 00 41 227339291

Brussels Secretariat:
74 Rue de Trèves
B-1040 Brussels
Belgium
Tel 00 322 2861711
Fax 00 322 2861750

The Council of Europe

Palais De l'Europe
F-67075 Strasbourg Cedex
France
Tel 00 33 88412000
Fax 00 33 88412781

World Health Organization

20 Avenue Appia	Regional Office for Europe
CH-1211	Scherfigsuj 8
Geneva 27	DK 2100
Switzerland	Copenhagen
Tel 00 41 227912111	Denmark
	Tel 00 45 39171717

The European Foundation for the Improvement of Living and Working Conditions

Loughlinstown House
Shankill
Co Dublin
Ireland
Tel 00 353 12826888
Fax 00 353 12826456

European Centre for the Development of Vocational Training (CEDEFOP)

CEDEFOP is an organization established by the Council of the European Community in 1975. It provides technical support to the Commission of the European Union and has information, research and consultation functions in the field of vocational training.

Marinou Antipa 12, GR-57001 Thessaloniki, Greece.
Tel 00 3031 490111
Fax 00 3031 490102

European Parliament Intergroup on Health

c/o European Public Health Alliance
1 Place du Luxembourg
B-1040 Brussels
Belgium
Tel 00 322 5129360
Fax 00 322 5126673

Organization for Economic Co-operation and Development (OECD)

2 Rue André-Pascal
75775 Paris Cedex 16
France
Tel 00 331 45248200
Fax 00 331 45248500

2. UK Government

UK Permanent Representatives to the Community (UKRep)

Rond Point Schuman 6
B-1040 Brussels
Belgium
Tel 00 322 2878211
Fax 00 322 2878398

House of Commons Select Committee on European Legislation

Overseas Office
House of Commons
London SW1A 0AA
Tel 0171 219 3292
Fax 0171 219 2509

(There is also a House of Lords European Communities Select Committee, with a sub-committee on the Environment, Public Health and Education.)

The Department of Health

Richmond House
79 Whitehall
London SW1A 2NS
Tel 0171 210 2020
Fax 0171 210 5523

The Department for Education and Employment

The Comparability Co-ordinator
Room E454
Moorfoot
Sheffield
S1 4PO
Tel 0114 2594144

3.   European health groups and professional associations

Many pan-European health care organizations exist, with varying degrees of influence in European matters. The following are a sample of the more active ones. For a more comprehensive list of such organizations, consult the *European Health Services Handbook*.

The European Public Health Alliance (EPHA)

1 Place du Luxembourg
B-1040 Brussels
Belgium
Tel 00 322 5129360
Fax 00 322 5126673

EPHA aims to: promote co-operation, monitor EC development in the health area; ensure that the health point of view is taken into account in all major EC policy areas; influence EC institutions and others; promote improve health status; provide a focus for discussion; and seek more systematic consultation of health associations within the Commission and other EC institutions.

The Hospital Committee of the European Community (HCEC)

Hospital Committee of the European Community
Kapucijnenvoer 35
3000 Leuven
Belgium
Tel 00 32 16216902
Fax 00 32 16216970

A non-governmental European association, HCEC includes national hospital associations as well as a representative from the national or regional health system of the Member States of the EU and Switzerland. It organizes and funds the HOPE exchange programme (referred to in Chapter 6) and is also currently collecting data on hospital and other health-related twinnings and has produced a glossary of hospital terminology used in the Member States. The UK representative is Sir William Doughty, Chairman of North West Thames RHA.

European Healthcare Management Association (EHMA)

The Director
EHMA
Vergemount Hall
Clonskeagh
Dublin 6
Ireland
Tel 00 353 1 2839299
Fax 00 353 1 2698644

An independent organization committed to developing managerial expertise in European health services by enhancing the quality and effectiveness of health care management, education, training and development.

The European Association of Hospital Managers (EAHM)

Secretary General: Claude-Guy Charlotte
Centre Hospitalier Regional
1 Place de l'Hôpital
67091 Strasbourg Cedex
France
Tel 00 33 88161150
Fax 00 33 88161330

EAHM is a non-profit making association representing national associations or groups of hospital managers in the EU. Its aim is to provide hospital services, in particular hospital management in European countries, by proposing new ideas, enabling the exchange of experience and exploiting the results of research undertaken in all relevant fields.

Association of Schools of Public Health in the European Region (ASPHER)

Bernard Junod
Ecole Nationale de la Santé Publique
Avenue du Professeur Leon Bernard
35043 Rennes Cedex
France
Tel 00 33 99282930
Fax 00 33 99282828

ASPHER provides a focus for the development of collaborative education and research activities in public health at a European level.

European Union of Medical Specialists (UEMS)

c/o GBS
20 Avenue de la Couronne
B-1050 Brussels
Belgium
Tel 00 322 6495164
Fax 00 322 6403730

European Health Policy Forum (EHPF)

1 Place du Luxembourg
B-1040 Brussels
Belgium
Tel 00 322 5129360
Fax 00 322 5126673

Although not a European association like those listed above, the London School of Economic's LSE Health initiative must be included here.

LSE Health

The London School of Economics and Political Science
Houghton Street
London WC2A 2AE
Tel 0171 9557540
Fax 0171 9557546

LSE Health conducts research and teaching in the health policy area, particularly within a European context, and advises governmental and non-governmental bodies.

4. Standing Committees

The Commission seeks views and opinions from various interest groups but also relies on a series of Standing Committees established through provisions made in previous Treaties. Addresses for two are given below:

Standing Committee of Doctors of the EC

66 Avenue de Cortenburgh, Bte 2
B-1040 Brussels
Belgium
Tel 00 322 7327202
Fax 00 322 7327344

Standing Committee of Nurses of the EC

34 Rue Leys
B-1040 Brussels
Belgium
Tel 00 322 7368029
Fax 00 322 7337862

Section B   Contracts for European programmes

Most EU programmes have a national contact or assistance unit as well as a Brussels-based (or Luxembourg-based) European contact, either in the European Commission or in a Technical Assistance Office. Wherever relevant, both of these have been provided, but it is best to approach the national contact first. This usually results in a more rapid response but also ensures that enquirers receive documentation which includes any priorities, eligibility criteria and details of UK contact points. (The programmes themselves are described in Chapter 7.)

1.   European Social Fund (ESF)

(NB: applications should be presented via eligible organizations supported by a public authority.)
'Mainstream' ESF general address:

European Social Fund Unit

Department for Education and Employment
236 Gray's Inn Road
London WC1X 8HL
Tel 0171 2114740
Fax 0171 2114749

Human Resource Community Initiatives

Employment NOW
Employment HORIZON
Employment YOUTHSTART
ADAPT

Lorraine Harris
European Social Fund Section
Department for Education and Employment
236 Gray's Inn Road
London WC1X 8HL
Tel 0171 211 4710/4740/4741
Fax 0171 2114749

General information on the Community Initiatives is available from:

Yvonne Corbett
DTI
European Cohesion Branch
Room 317
3.A.49
1 Victoria Street
London SW1H 0ET
Tel 0171 2152557

2. Education and training programmes

Leonardo da Vinci
Different sections of the Department for Education and Employment deal with different strands of the programme. General enquiries can be addressed to:

European Training Branch
Department for Education and Employment
Room 513
Steel House
Tothill Street
London SW1H 9NF
Tel 0171 2735406
Fax 0171 2735475

Brussels contact:
Leonardo Technical Assistance Office
9 Avenue de l'Astronomie
B-1030 Brussels
Belgium
Tel 00 322 2270100
Fax 00 322 2270101

Socrates
There are different contacts for the various programme strands.

Higher education:
The Erasmus Grants Council
The University
Canterbury
Kent
CT2 7PD
Tel 01227 762712

Lingua and **Comenius** are split between the Central Bureau and the Department for Education and Employment. For more information contact:

The Central Bureau for Educational Visits and Exchanges
Seymour Mews House
Seymour Mews
London WIH 9PE
Tel 0171 3894004 (general switchboard)
Fax 0171 2241906

Brussels contact:
Socrates and Youth Technical Assistance Office
70 Rue Montoyer
B-1040 Brussels
Belgium
Tel 00 322 2330111
Fax 00 322 2330150

3.   Research and development

Biotechnology (Biotech II)
UK contacts:
Dr Alf Game
Biotechnology and Biological Research Centre
Polaris House
North Star Avenue
Swindon SN2 1EU
Tel 01793 413354
Fax 01793 413382
and
Liz Hawken
DTI
Chemicals and Biotechnology Division
Laboratory of the Government Chemist
Queens Road
Teddington
Middlesex TW11 0LY
Tel 0181 9437338
Fax 0181 9437304

European Commission responsible person:
Etienne Magnien
DGXII/E-1
European Commission
200 Rue de la Loi
B-1049 Brussels
Belgium
Tel 00 322 2959347
Fax 00 322 2955365

Biomedicine and Health (Biomed II)

UK contact:
Mrs Gillian Breen
Medical Research Council
20 Park Crescent
London WIN 4AL
Tel 0171 6365422
Fax 0171 4366179

European Commission responsible person:
Andre Emmanuel Baert
DGXII
European Commission
200 Rue de la Loi
B-1049 Brussels
Belgium
Tel 00 322 2958647
Fax 00 322 2955365

Telematics programmes

Health Care (formerly known as AIM)
UK contacts:
David Preston
Department of Health
5th Floor
Quarry House
Quarry Hill
Leeds LS2 7UE
Tel 0113 2546003
Fax 0113 2546030

and
Brian Jones
DTI
151 Buckingham Palace Road
London SW1W 9SS
Tel 0171 2151224
Fax 0171 2151370

European Commission responsible person:
Prof. Jean-Claude Healey
DGXIII/C
European Commission
200 Rue de la Loi
B-1049 Brussels
Belgium
Tel 00 322 2963506
Fax 00 322 2960181

Elderly and Disabled (TIDE)

UK contacts:
Dr Tony Shipley
Medical Devices Directorate
Department of Health
Room 313
13–16 Russell Square
London WC1B 5EP
Tel 0171 9728180
Fax 0171 9728106
and
Brian Jones
DTI
Palace Street
London SW1E 5HE
Tel 0171 2382763
Fax 0171 2382793

European Commission responsible person:
Egidio Ballabio
DGXIII/C
European Commission

Rue de la Loi 200
B-1049 Brussels
Belgium
Tel 00 322 2990232
Fax 00 322 2990248

4. Public health programmes

(Applications are made direct to DGV of the Commission.)

Health promotion

DGV/F/3
European Commission
Bâtiment Jean Monnet
Plateau du Kirchberg
L-2920 Luxembourg
Tel 00 352 430132007
Fax 00 352 430134511

Europe Against Cancer

Mme Soledad Blanco
DGV/F
Bâtiment Jean Monnet
Plateau du Kirchberg
L-2920 Luxembourg
Tel 00 352 430137324
Fax 00 352 43013475

AIDS and communicable diseases

Dr H. Martin
DGV/F/2
Bâtiment Jean Monnet
Plateau du Kirchberg
L-2920 Luxembourg
Tel 00 352 430132738

Section C   Information networks: European Documentation Centres, Euro Info Centres and EURES Euro-advisers in the UK

There are several information networks on EU matters in the UK, in addition to whatever local and regional information services may have been established by local authorities and other interested groups, and the public library service. The first of these to be set up were the **European Documentation Centres** (EDCs), which are usually (but not invariably) based in the libraries of academic institutions, though open to the general public. Some cities (Birmingham, Coventry and Leeds) have two EDCs and there are several in London. Most EDCs offer reference facilities only (i.e. material is not available on loan) and do not have sufficient staff to offer an advice service or detailed assistance with enquiries.

Aberdeen

European Documentation Centre
Aberdeen University Library
Queen Mother Library
Meston Walk
Aberdeen AB9 2UE, UK
Tel (44–224) 27 25 88
Fax (44–224) 48 70 48

Bath

University of Bath
University Library
Bath BA2 7AY
Tel (44–225) 82 68 26 Ext 5594
Fax (44–225) 82 62 29

Belfast

The Queen's University of Belfast
Main Library
Government Publications Dept
Belfast BT7 1LS
Tel (44–232) 24 51 33 Ext 3605
Fax (44–232) 32 33 40

Birmingham

European Documentation Centre
Information Service
Perry Barr Library
University of Central England in Birmingham
Birmingham B42 2SU

University of Birmingham
Official Publications Dept
Main Library
PO Box 363
Birmingham B15 2TT
Tel (44–21) 414 58 23

Bradford

The Librarian
University of Bradford
Richmond Road
Bradford BD7 1DP
Tel (44–1274) 38 34 02/73 34 66 Ext 3402
Fax (44–1274) 38 33 98

Bristol

The University of Bristol
Law & Geology Libraries
and European Documentation Centre
Wills Memorial Building
Queen's Road
Bristol BS8 1RJ
Tel (44–117) 928 79 44

Cambridge

Librarian, Cambridge University Library
West Road
Cambridge CB3 9DR
Tel (44–223) 33 31 38
Fax (44–223) 33 31 60

Canterbury

The University of Kent at Canterbury
European Documentation Centre
The Library
Canterbury, Kent CT2 7NU
Tel (44–227) 76 40 00 Ext 31 09

Cardiff

Arts & Social Studies Library
Official Publ. Librarian
European Documentation Centre
University of Wales
College of Cardiff
PO Box 430
Cardiff CF1 3XT
Tel (44–206) 871 31

Co. Londonderry

University of Ulster
European Documentation Centre
Library
Cromore Road
Coleraine
Co. Londonderry BT52 1S
Tel (44–265) 41 41 Ext 4257
Fax (44–265) 555 13

Colchester

University of Essex
Library-EDC
PO Box 24
Colchester CO4 3UA
Tel (44–206) 87 33 33
Fax (44–206) 87 35 98

Coventry

European Documentation Centre
Lanchester Library
Coventry University

Much Park Street
Coventry CV1 2HF
Tel (44–203) 83 84 52/83 86 98

The University of Warwick
European Documentation Centre
Periodicals Dept
The Library
Coventry CV4 7AL
Tel (02–03) 52 30 33/52 35 23 Ext 2041

Dundee

The University of Dundee
Faculty of Law
The Library
Dundee DD1 4HN
Tel (44–382) 231 81 Ext 4100

Durham

University of Durham
Official Publications Collection
University Library
Stockton Road
Durham DH1 3LY
Tel (44–91)374 30 41/4

Edinburgh

Europa Library
Librarian
University of Edinburgh
Old College
South Bridge
Edinburgh EH8 9YL
Tel (44–31) 650 20 41/667 10 11 Ext 4292
Fax (44–31) 667 79 38

Exeter

The Librarian
European Documentation Centre
Exeter University Law Library

Amory Building
Rennes Drive
Exeter EX4 4RJ
Tel (44–392) 26 33 56
Fax (44–392) 26 31 08

Falmer, Brighton

European Documentation Centre
Documents Section
University of Sussex Library
Falmer, Brighton BN1 9QL
Tel (44–273) 67 81 59

Glasgow

University of Glasgow
The Library
Hillhead Street
Glasgow G12 8QE
Tel (44–41) 339 88 55 Ext 67 44
Fax (44–41) 357 50 43

Guildford

European Documentation Centre
George Edwards Library
University of Surrey
Guildford, Surrey GU2 5XH
Tel (44–1483) 25 92 33
Fax (44–1483) 25 95 00

Hull

The University of Hull
Brynmor Jones Library
European Documentation Centre
Cottingham Road
Hull HU6 7RX
Tel (44–482) 46 54 11

Keele

The Librarian
University of Keele

European Documentation Centre
Keele, Staffordshire ST5 5BG
Tel (44–782) 62 11 11 Ext 3738
Fax (44–782) 61 38 47

Lancaster

University of Lancaster
Serials Section
University Library
Lancaster LA1 4YH
Tel (44–524) 652 01 Ext 276
Fax (44–524) 638 06

Leeds

Leeds Metropolitan University Library
European Documentation Centre
Calverley Street
Leeds LS1 3HE
Tel (44–113) 283 31 26
Fax (44–113) 283 31 23

University of Leeds
European Documentation Centre
Faculty of Law
20 Lyddon Terrace
Leeds LS2 9JT
Tel (44–532) 33 50 40/33 55 12

Leicester

Leicester University Library
European Documentation Centre
PO Box 248
University Road
Leicester LE1 9QD
Tel (44–533) 52 20 44
Fax (44–533) 52 20 66

London

European Documentation Centre
Library and Information Service

University of North London
1 Prince of Wales Road
London NW5 3LB
Tel (44–71) 753 51 42/607 27 89 Ext 4110
Fax (44–71) 753 50 78

Information Production Group
National Association of Citizen's Advice Bureaux
115–123 Pentonville Road
London N1 9LZ

International Organisation Collection
London School of Economics
EDC/British Library of Political and Economic Science
10 Portugal Street
London WC2A 2HD
Tel (44–71) 955 72 73
Fax (44–71) 955 74 54

Local Government International Bureau
35 Great Smith Street
London SW1P 3BJ
Tel (44–71) 222 16 36
Fax (44–71) 233 21 79

Librarian
Trades Union Congress
Congress House
Great Russel Street
London WC1B 3LS

The Library
University of London
Queen Mary and Westfield College
Mile End Road
London E1 4NS
Tel (44–71) 975 55 55
Fax (44–71) 975 55 00

The Royal Institute of International Affairs Library
Chatham House
10 St James's Square

London SW1Y 4LE
Tel (44–71) 957 57 21
Fax (44–71) 957 57 10

Loughborough

University of Technology
Pilkington Library
Serials Office
Loughborough, Leicestershire LE11 3TU
Tel (44–509) 22 23 44

Manchester

Manchester University
Europ. Documentation Centre
John Rylands University
Library
Miss S. J. Clarke (for the Assistant Librarian)
Oxford Road
Manchester M13 9PP
Tel (44–61) 273 74 88
Fax (44–61) 275 37 64/51

Newcastle upon Tyne

The University of Northumbria at Newcastle
Library
Europ. Documentation Centre
Ellison Building
Ellison Place
Newcastle upon Tyne NE1 8ST
Tel (44–91) 235 81 36
Fax (44–91) 261 69 11

Norwich

University of East Anglia
The Library
University Plain
Norwich NR4 7TJ
Tel (44–603) 561 61 Ext 2412
Fax (44–603) 25 94 90

Nottingham

Nottingham University
University Library
Nottingham NG7 2RD
Tel (44–602) 48 48 48 Ext 3741

Oxford

The Bodleian Law Library
University of Oxford
European Documentation Centre
Manor Road
Oxford OX1 3UR
Tel (44–865) 27 14 63
Fax (44–865) 27 14 75

Portsmouth

Periodicals Section
Portsmouth Polytechnic
Library
Cambridge Road
Portsmouth PO1 2ST
Tel (44–705) 82 76 81 Ext 3240

Reading

The Library
European Documentation Centre
University of Reading
Whiteknights
PO Box 223
Reading RG6 2AE
Tel (44–734) 31 87 82
Fax (44–734) 31 23 35

Salford

EDC Librarian
Clifford Whitworth
University Library
Salford, Lancashire M5 4WT
Tel (44–61) 745 50 00 Ext 3662

Sheffield

European Documentation Centre
Library
Sheffield Polytechnic
Pond Street
Sheffield S1 1WB
Tel (44–742) 72 09 11

Southampton

Periodicals Dept.
University Library
Southampton University
Southampton, Hants SO9 5NH
Tel (44–902) 55 90 00

Wolverhampton

Robert Scott Library
University of Wolverhampton
St Peter's Square
Wolverhampton WV1 1RH
Tel (44–902) 31 30 05 Ext 2300/32 10 00

Wye, Ashford

The Library
Wye College
Wye, Ashford, Kent TN25 5A
Tel (44–233) 81 24 01 Ext 497

For those wanting a little more in the way of help, one of the best sources of information and advice on European Union matters is the network of **Euro Info Centres** or EICs. These were originally established with the business community in mind, and specifically, small and medium sized enterprises (SMEs) but are actually consulted by a wide range of organizations. They are linked by on-line databases and have staff who are specially trained to deal with EU information enquiries. EICs may charge a small fee to cover their costs. Many enquiries are processed by telephone or fax.

Euro Info Centre Limited
21 Bothwell Street
Glasgow G2 6NL
Tel 041 221 0999
Fax 041 221 6539
Contact: **Ian Traill**

Euro Info Centre
Birmingham Chamber of Commerce & Industry
75 Harbourne Road
PO Box 360
Birmingham B15 3DH
Tel 0121 454 6171
Fax 0121 455 8670
Contact: **Cathy Davies**

Euro Info Centre
Northern Development Company
Great North House
Sandyford Road
Newcastle upon Tyne NE1 8ND
Tel 0191 261 0026/5131
Fax 0191 222 1774
Contact: **Marion Schooler**

Euro Info Centre
Local Enterprise Development Unit
(LEDU)
Ledu House
Upper Galwally
Belfast BT8 4TB
Tel 01232 49 1031
Fax 01232 69 1432
Contact: **Eleanor Butterwick**

Euro Info Centre
Sussex Chamber of Commerce and Industry
169 Church Road
Hove BN3 2AS
Tel 01273 326282
Fax 01273 207965
Contact: **Vivienne Gray**

Euro Info Centre
Bristol Chamber of Commerce and Industry
16 Clifton Park
Bristol BS8 3BY
Tel 01272 737373
Fax 01272 745365
Contact: **Sarah Harris**

Euro Info Centre Southwest
Exeter Enterprises
Reed Hall
University of Exeter
Exeter EX4 4QR
Tel 01392 214085
Fax 01392 264375
Contact: **Diana Letcher**

Euro Info Centre
European Business Services
Business Information Source
20 Bridge Street
Inverness IV1 1QR
Tel 01463 715400/702560
Fax 01463 715600
Contact: **Caroline Gray-Stephens**

Humberside European Business Information Centre (HEBIC)
University of Hull
Brynmor Jones Library
Hull HU6 7RX
Tel 01482 465940/35
Fax 01482 466488
Contact: **Sally Hewitt**

Euro Info Centre
Leicester European Information Centre
The Business Centre
10 York Road
Leicester LE1 5TS
Tel 01533 559944
Fax 01533 553470
Contact: **Rita Ganata**

Euro Info Centre North West
Liverpool Central Libraries
William Brown Street
Liverpool L3 8EW
Tel 0151 298128
Fax 0151 2071342
e-mail dawn@eicnw.u-net.com
Contact: **Howard Patterson**

Kent European Information Centre
County Council Economic Development Unit
Springfield
Maidstone ME14 2LL
Tel 01622 694109
Fax 01622 691418
Contact: **David Oxlade**

Manchester Euro Info Centre
Business Link Manchester
Churchgate House
56 Oxford Street
Manchester M60 7BL
Tel 0161 2374190/4020
Fax 0161 2369945
Contact: **Peter Maher**

Euro Info Centre
Norfolk and Waveney Chamber of Commerce and Industry
112 Barrack Street
Norwich NR3 1UB
Tel 01603 625977
Fax 01603 633032
Contact: **Sarah Abercrombie**

Euro Info Centre
Nottingham Chamber of Commerce and Industry
309 Haydn Road
Nottingham NG5 1DG
Tel 01602 624624
Fax 01602 856612
Contact: **Graham Birkett**

Wales Euro Info Centre
UWCC – Guest Building
PO Box 430
Cardiff CF1 3XT
Tel 01222 229525
Fax 01222 229740
e-mail cw63@CityScape.co.uk/wilcoxb@cardiff.ac.uk
Contact: **Brian Wilcox**

Wales Euro Info Centre
Library & Information Services
County Civic Centre
Mold CH7 6NW
Tel 01352 704748
Fax 01352 753662
Contact: **Eric Davies**

Thames Valley Euro Info Centre
Commerce House
2–6 Bath Road
Slough SL1 3SB
Tel 01753 577877
Fax 01753 524644
Contact: **Mark Sharman**

Shropshire and Staffordshire Euro Info Centre
Trevithick House
4 Stafford Park
Telford TF3 3BA
Tel 01952 208213/228
Fax 01952 208208
Contact: **Susan Johnson**

Euro Info Centre Southern Area
Civic Centre
Southampton SO9 4XP
Tel 01703 832866
Fax 01703 231714
Contact: **David Dance**

Euro Info Centre
West Yorkshire European Business Information Centre
(WYEBIC)

4 Manchester Road
Mercury House – 2nd Floor
Bradford BD5 0QL
Tel 01274 754262
Fax 01274 393226
Contact: **Jenny Lawson**

Mid-Yorkshire Euro Info Centre
Leeds Metropolitan University Library
Calverley Street
Leeds LS1 3HE
Tel 0113 2833126
Fax 0113 2833123
Contact: **Meg Message**

Staffordshire European Business Centre
Staffordshire Development Association
Shire Hall
Market Street
Stafford ST16 2LQ
Tel 01785 59528
Fax 01785 215286
Contact: **Tim Hiscock**

Euro Info Centre
London Chamber of Commerce and Industry
33 Queen Street
London EC4R 1AP
Tel 0171 489 1992
Fax 0171 489 0391
Contact: **Beth Rayney-Cucala**

More recently, public libraries have been encouraged to act as **Public Information Relay** centres. These hold a stock of reference documents and are only able to deal with personal callers, rather than telephone enquiries. Staff may refer enquirers to another source of information if they are unable to provide the assistance required. The Relay centres are not distributed equally around the UK and some readers may find they have no service in their town or city because the library service there has not become involved. If this is the case, it is still worth checking with local libraries in case they still offer an information service on European matters; if no service is provided, lobbying local councillors may have results.

The service offered by the network of **Euroadvisers** is more specialized, and focuses on employment and work-related information. Euroadvisers offer services to employers seeking to recruit and also to job seekers (unemployed or not), and provide not only information about practical recruitment and employment matters but general information on living and working in another country. For those intending to make a move, or simply seeking to explore the possibilities, their services are an essential first step. A list of telephone numbers for the UK Euroadvisers is provided below:

Belfast:	Oonagh McDonnell, 01232 252270 (Training and Employment Agency)
Birmingham:	Lyndley Jenks, 0121 4525409 (Employment Service)
Bristol:	Rosemary Bird, 0117 9456730 (Employment Service)
Cardiff:	Sheila Pithouse, 01222 380780 (Employment Service)
Eastbourne:	Leslie Ford, 01323 737317 (SERTUC)
Edinburgh:	Colin Mills, 0131 5569211 (Employment Service)
Leeds:	Joanne Woodhead, 0113 2459546 (Employment Service)
London:	Stephen Fletcher, 0171 2114912 and Margaret Toale, 0171 2114320 (Employment Service)
Manchester:	Helen Langdon, 0161 8731225 (Employment Service)
Newcastle:	Christopher Thwaites, 0191 2114401 (Employment Service)
Nottingham:	Allison Clark, 0115 9483308 (Employment Service)
Omagh:	John McKay, 01662 244921 (Training and Employment Agency)
Sheffield:	Terry Caine, 0114 2596086 and Ian Foulstone, 0114 2596089 (Employment Service Head Office)

Section D   Useful publications (including on-line information)

There are far too many publications about the European Union to list in full. A short selection of the most useful and relevant, both generally and to the field of health care, is provided in the following pages (and in the recommended reading suggested at the end of chapters). Many more exist and readers are recommended to visit their local EDCs/EICs to view a wide range.

1. General

Numerous publications are produced by the European Commission, and perhaps the most readable regular digest of issues and events is *The Week in Europe*, a weekly bulletin sent out by the Storey's Gate Press Office. It is usually no more than 2 sides of A4, summarizing the main events and developments of the past week. In addition, the Commission publishes *Background Reports* on a range of topical issues and developments. Both of these are free but Commission staff will not take requests for them over the phone, so organizations or individuals must write to the London office and ask to be put on the mailing list.

A range of other publications are available from the DGs or the Commission Publications Office. A useful general bulletin is: *Eur-Op News*, Information from the European Communities Publications Office (free of charge) – published four times a year.

Contact:
Eur-Op News
Office 172
2 Rue Mercier
L 2985 Luxembourg or fax 00 352 292942763

The European Commission is actually a considerable publisher in its own right; a list of publications can be requested from regional offices in the UK. Centrally, its Luxembourg office also produces the most important primary source document, *The Official Journal of the European Communities*. The 'L'

(Legislation) and 'C' (Information and Notices) series are the most informative, with other separate series dealing with public contracts (the Supplement). Subscriptions are via HMSO (Her Majesty's Stationery Office) but the 'OJs' are easily accessible via EDCs and EICs.

Apart from Commission-produced material, the most useful digest of EU issues for those working in the public sector is produced by the Local Government International Bureau. The European Information Service (EIS) is tailored specifically to the needs of those in local government but provides an excellent overview of a range of issues (including health) of interest to public sector-based workers and organizations. EIS is in ten issues per annum. (There is a subscription charge, so check it out in the library before making a commitment.)

Address:
35 Great Smith Street, London SE1P 3PJ
Tel 0171 222 1636
Fax 0171 233 2179

In addition to the above, there are a range of guides produced by private sector companies, some loose leaf formats with regular updates (e.g. EUROFI), others smaller booklets. They are usually available on annual subscriptions. One example is *Vacher's European Companion and Consultants' Register*.

Address:
Vachers' Publications
113 High Street
Berkhamstead
Herts HP4 2DJ
Tel 01442 876135

Again, check these out in the library or ask for a sample copy before deciding to subscribe.

Some professional associations and institutes also produce their own European newsletters. One example is the **Institute of Personnel Management's** *European Community Update*, a monthly brief on EC Developments in the employment field. Aimed at personnel professionals, it has covered the Social

Charter Action programme, EC employment law cases and other EC developments in the areas of health and safety, equality, training, free movement and employment generally.

Contact:
IPM House
Camp Road
Wimbledon
London SW19 4UX

2. Health care publications

Public health and the EU: an overview
A4 sized booklet produced by EPHA, the European Public Health Alliance (see earlier section for address). EPHA also produces *European Public Health Update*, available monthly by subscription, and an extremely well-focused and useful bulletin.

Echo – Health and Social Services in Europe and Overseas
A Department of Health newsletter, published nine times a year by NHS Publicity Service on behalf of the Department of Health International Relations Unit. Distribution enquiries contact:
Lorna Demming 0171 972 2330

Euro Med Info
Monthly reports on European Community initiatives in the field of pharmaceutical and health. Copies are available from:
John Stephenson
Euro Med Info
Mc: Medical and Media Communications
Brigade House
8 Parsons Green
London
SW6 4TN
Tel 0171 371 5044

3. Books and reference material

Note: HMSO Books (Agency Section) are the UK sales agents for all European Union publications. If you have difficulty obtaining any EU publication, contact HMSO Publications Centre, 51 Nine Elms Lane, London SW85 5DR.

European Health Services Handbook
by N. Leadbeater. Published on behalf of EHMA, IHSM and NAHAT by the Institute of Health Service Management, London, 1993.

The Directory of Higher Education Institutions provides the addresses of 4000 higher learning institutions in the EU, together with indexed information on the subject and occupational areas in which they award diplomas (co-published by EUR-OP and Kogan Page).

Working in France, Spain, etc. available from:
Employment Service Overseas Placing Unit
Steel House
Moorfoot
Sheffield S1 4PQ.

The EU Inter-Institutional Yearbook. This contains all the names of the heads of units, their postal addresses, a list of buildings where all the EU institutions are housed, etc. This directory will enable users to identify appropriate administrators and decision-makers (obtainable from HMSO, Cat. No. CB 87 95 353).

The Central Bureau for Educational Visits and Exchanges produces a number of publications, including *Seasonal Jobs*, *Voluntary Work* and *Language Courses*, available from:
The Central Bureau
Seymour Mews
London W1H 9PE.

EUROSTAT publications are designed both to inform readers of statistics through tables, selected commentaries and illustrations, and to steer them towards more specialized sources. The EUROSTAT catalogue appears annually and is available from the EUROSTAT office or EUR-OP.

Social Europe is a twice-yearly publication which is a useful source of information on measures taken in the European social field. It is available by annual subscription from either HMSO or the Office for Official Publications of the EU. Single copies can also be ordered. In addition, there are four or five supplements each year on specific issues, plus *Social Europe Magazine*, which is published every four months.

Journal of European Social Policy
Longman Higher Educational Journals
Longman House
Burnt Mill
Harlow
Essex CM20 2JE.

European Journal of Public Health
Oxford University Press.

Le Magazine. A free newsletter which provides information on education and training issues. Published by DGXXII of the European Commission. To be included on the mailing list, write to the European Commission in Brussels or fax a request to 00 322 2957295.

The European Hospital. Published by Beta Publishing
Hong-Kong Ltd
Room 1201
Dina House
11 Duddle Street
Central Hong Kong.

Euroforum. Produced quarterly by the Royal College of Nursing.
20 Cavendish Square
London
W1M 0AB.

Janus is a free newsletter dealing with the problems of health and safety at work. Published by DGV.
The European Commission
L 2929 Luxembourg.

Helioscope/Helios Flash is a European Commission disability magazine which reports regularly on developments in European social and employment policy of interest to disabled people and those who work with them.

Eurohealth

The Health Policy Research Network and LSE Health
London School of Economics
Houghton Street
London WC2A 2AE.

Society & Health

The King's Fund Policy Institute
11–13 Cavendish Square
London W1M 0AN.

International Healthcare News

Available from: FT Pharmaceuticals & Healthcare Publishing
Via-Aura House
53 Oldridge Road
London SW12 8PJ

European Hospital Management Journal.

Olive Tree Publishing Ltd
15 Berners Street
London W1P 3DE.

New Directory of Public Databases: the fourth edition includes descriptions of 44 databases produced by the EU Commission, by other EU institutions and EUR-OP. It contains information on the distribution organizations, including distributors of CD-ROMs and diskettes (contact EUR-OP).

Hospital Services in the EC – Organisation and Terminology
Hospital Committee of the European Community (1993)
Kapucijnenvoer 35
B-3000 Leuven
Brussels
Belgium.

Networking in the European Union.
Royal College of Nursing, 1994.

4. Databases and on-line information

The Commission is committed to encouraging the development of an information society and is making as much material as possible available via on line databases, CD-ROM, and more recently, the Internet. DGX, the section of the Commission responsible for information, is linked to the Internet via the **Europa** server pilot project. Europa contains general information on the EU, an ABC of policies and information on how to access the Commission's databases, such as **Cordis** and **Eurostat**. The access code for Europa is http://www.cec.lu.

Information on individual databases can be obtained from EUR-OP (the Office for Official Publications) in Luxembourg. Tel 00 352 292942455, Fax 00 352 292942763.

5. Videos and teaching aids

EUR-OP produces a catalogue of videos (for the address, see above, or contact HMSO). Other useful materials are the Education Europe 2000 European information modules, also available on CD-ROM.

Contact:
Director of Publications
Education 2000
7a Westminster Street
Yeovil
Somerset BA20 1AF.

Part 3

Select glossary of terms and 'Eurojargon'

N.B. this is not an exhaustive list.

ACSTT   Advisory Committee on Scientific and Technical Training

ADAPT   One of the Community Initiatives group of programmes running from 1994–99, the aim of ADAPT is to assist the adaptation of the European workforce to industrial and technological change.

ALTENER   Alternative Energy programme

AIM   Advanced Informatics in Medicine (now Telematics for Healthcare).

AMUE   Association for the Monetary Union of Europe

ASEAN   Association of South East Asian countries linked to the EU – Malaysia, Indonesia Philippines, Singapore, Thailand and Brunei.

Avicienne Initiative   Programme aimed at exploring possibilities for scientific and technical co-operation via joint research projects on a shared cost basis, between EU Member States and Mediterranean countries, in three designated areas, one being primary health care.

BC-NET   Business Co-operation Network – computer-based network linking business advisers throughout the EU and in other non-member countries.

BECU   Billion ECU

BEUC   European Consumers' Organisation

BIC   Business and Information centres

BIOMED   now BIOMED II, part of the Fourth Framework Programme for Research and

	Technological Development, and a programme to assist transnational research into health-related problems.
BIOTECH	Again, part of the Fourth Framework Programme. BIOTECH II concentrates on a number of areas such as genome analysis, immunology, etc.
BRAIN	Basic Research in Adaptive Intelligence and Neuro-computing
BRIC	Biotechnology Regulations Inter-service Communities
BRIDGE	Biotechnology Research for Innovation, Development Growth in Europe
BRITE/EURAM	Basic Research in Industrial Technologies in Europe/European Research on Advanced Materials
CAP	Common Agricultural Policy
CCC	Consumers' Consultative Committee of the EEC
CEC	Commission of the European Communities
CEDEFOP	European Centre for Vocational Training (based in Thessaloniki).
CEFIC	European Chemical Industry Council (based in Brussels).
CELAD	Co-ordinators' Group on Drugs
CEN	European Committee for Standardisation
CEPS	Centre for European Policy Studies – independent research institute, established in 1983 to encourage the study of public affairs. Based in Brussels.
College of Europe	Institution founded in 1949 in Bruges. It offers one-year European studies programmes to graduates.
CERD	European Research and Development Committee
CERN	European Organisation for Nuclear Research (another CERN is the European laboratory for Particle Physics).
CFP	Common Fisheries Policy

CIAA	Confederation of the Food and Drink Industries of the EC
CIDST	Committee for Scientific and Technical Information and Documentation
CIRCE	Centre for EC Information and Documentary Research
COMECON	Council for Mutual Economic Assistance
CODEST	Committee for the Development of Science and Technology
CoE	Council of Europe
COFACE	Confederation of Family Organisations in the EC (based in Brussels).
COMETT	Community Action Programme for Education and Training for Technology
CORDIS	Community Research and Development Information Service (see contact/information section).
COREPER	Committee of Permanent Representatives, made up of ambassadors from the Member States to the European Union.
COST	European Co-operation in Science and Technology
CRAFT	An EU RTD programme entitled Co-operative Research Action for Technology
CREST	Scientific and Technical Research Committee (administered by DGXII).
CRM	Committee for Medical and Public Health Research
CSF	Community Support Framework
CUBE	Concertation Unit for Biotechnology in Europe
DELTA	EU programme for Developing European Learning Through Technological Advance (now Area 4 of the RTD Telematics programmes, Flexible and Distance Education and Training).
ECHO	European Commission Host Organisation (on-line databases).
ECHO	European Community Humanitarian Office
ECFI	European Court of First Instance

ECJ	European Court of Justice
ECOFIN	Economic and Finance Council of Ministers
ECOS	European Cities Co-operation System
ECOSOC	Economic and Social Committee
ECSC	European Coal and Steel Community
ECU	European Currency Unit
EDC	European Documentation Centre
EEC	European Economic Community
EEIG	European Economic Interest Grouping
EES	European Economic Space
EFTA	European Free Trade Association
EIB	European Investment Bank
EIC	European Information Centre
EMEA	New European Agency for the Evaluation of Medicinal Products, based at Canary Wharf in London.
EMF	European Monetary Fund
EMU	European Monetary Union
ERASMUS	European Action Scheme for the Mobility of University Students
ERDF	European Regional Development Fund (also known by its French acronym, **FEDER**).
ERM	Exchange Rate Mechanism
ESPRIT	European Strategic Programme for Research and Technological Development in Information Technology
ETUC	European Trade Union Confederation
EUREKA	European Research Co-ordination Agency – launched in 1985 to encourage cross-border collaboration in research and technology between European countries (not solely EU). Now involves a number of eastern European countries.
EURES	European employment information network, to help job seekers in the EU find work in other Member States and also to help businesses recruit.
EURYDICE	Education Information Network in the EC

HANDYNET European information system in relation to disabled people – linked to HELIOS.

HELIOS Programme supporting best practice, etc. in relation to Handicapped People in the EU Living Independently in a Open Society

HORIZON One of the Community Initiatives programmes, and designed to improve the employment prospects of disadvantaged and disabled people.

INTERREG Now INTERREG II, a programme intended to assist cross-border co-operation, specifically for those internal and external border areas of the EU.

INTERPRISE Initiative to Encourage Partnerships between Industres and/or Services in Europe – aimed at SMEs and designed to stimulate co-operation.

IRDAC Industrial Research and Development Advisory Committee

ISPO Information Society Project Office

JOULE EU programme on Joint Opportunities for Unconventional or Long Term Energy Supply

KONVER Programme to assist regions which were formerly dependent on the defence industry and have been adversely affected by military spending cuts.

Leonardo da Vinci Umbrella programme which brings together five previous separate programmes dealing with training. Leonardo aims to bring a European dimension into training programmes, to encourage transnational developments and to support and complement the actions of Member State governments.

LIFE Programme for the environment.

LINGUA Originally a separate programme in its own right to promote language learning in

	the EU; now subsumed into Socrates and Leonardo.
MECU	Million ECU
MISEP	Mutual Information System on Employment Policies
MONITOR	Programme which is intended to identify new priorities for EU research and development.
NOW	Community Initiative programme aiming to reduce women's unemployment and improve the position of women in the workplace.
OECD	Organisation for Economic Co-operation and Development. Founded in 1961, its forerunner being the Organisation for European Economic Co-operation. Members include most EU countries and some which are not EU members, plus Japan, the US, Canada, Australia and New Zealand. Aims are to promote economic and social welfare of members and stimulate efforts to help developing countries.
OJ	*Official Journal*
OUVERTURE	Programme to encourage partnerships between regions and cities of the EU and Central and Eastern Europe, for transnational projects.
PHARE	Originally stood for Poland and Hungary: Assistance for Regeneration of the Economy. Now includes many other countries in need of technical and financial assistance.
RACE	Research and Development in Advanced Communications Technologies and Europe.
RECHAR	Programme to assist areas affected by the contraction of the coal industry.
RESIDER	Like the RECHAR programme, this programme aims to assist economic regeneration but of areas affected by the

contraction of the steel industry. (The RETEX programme is a similar initiative for the textile industry.)

Socrates Flagship programme for education, it aims to encourage innovation and improve quality in education by encouraging European co-operation and partnerships and assisting the integration of a European dimension. Sister programme to Leonardo.

STRIDE Science and Technology for Regional Innovation and Development in Europe

TACIS Technical Assistance for Economic Reform in the Commonwealth of Independent States and Georgia. Aimed at the countries of the former Soviet Union.

TED Tenders Electronic Daily – on-line database of European tenders.

TEMPUS Trans-European Mobility Programme for University Students

TIDE Technology Initiative for the Disabled and Elderly

UETP University Enterprise Training Programme

UNICE Union of Industrial and Employers' Confederation of Europe

URBAN One of the Community Initiatives, the URBAN programme is intended to help identify solutions to socio-economic problems experienced by urban areas.

VALUE Exploitation and Utilisation of Research Results in Europe

White Paper A document which sets out policies and intended action in a particular field or area of activity. It is often preceded by a Green Paper which is published as a consultative document. The ideas put forward in the Green Paper may be modified during consultation, or diluted. The White Paper is the blueprint for action.

YOUTHSTART   New Community initiatives programme which aims to encourage the integration of young people below the age of 20 into the workforce.

Index